Orthopaedic Neurology

ORTHOPAEDIC NEUROLOGY

A Diagnostic Guide to Neurologic Levels

Stanley Hoppenfeld, M.D.

Associate Clinical Professor of Orthopaedic Surgery and Director of
Scoliosis Service, Albert Einstein College of Medicine; Deputy
Director of Orthopaedic Surgery and Attending Physician, Bronx
Municipal Hospital Center; Associate Attending, Hospital for Joint Diseases
New York, New York

In collaboration with

Richard Hutton

Medical Illustrations by

Hugh Thomas

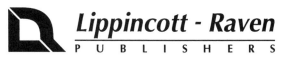

Lippincott - Raven
P U B L I S H E R S

Philadelphia • New York

ISBN 0-397-50368-7

Library of Congress Catalog Number 77-9316

Printed in the United States of America

30 29 28 27 26 25 24 23 22

Library of Congress Cataloging-in-Publication Data

Hoppenfeld, Stanley.
    Orthopaedic neurology.
    Bibliography: p.
    Includes index.
    1. Spinal cord—Diseases—Diagnosis.   2. Spinal cord—wounds and injuries—Diagnosis.
3. Nerves, Spinal Diseases—Diagnosis.   4. Nerves, Spinal Wounds and injuries—Diagnosis.
I. Hutton, Richard, joint author.   II. Title.   III. Title: Neurologic levels.
[DNLM: 1. Spinal cord diseases—Diagnosis.   2. Central nervous system diseases—Diagnosis.
3. Neurologic examination. WL300 H7980]

RC400.H66   616.8'3   77-9316
ISBN 0-397-50368-7

To My Family

Preface

Years ago I felt the need for a manual that would reduce the diagnosis of neurologic levels to its common denominators, and combine them with the basic principles of neurology to assist in the appraisal of spinal cord and nerve root problems. As the book began to take shape in my mind, it became apparent that the most important aspects of transmitting this information would lie in its organization and the clarity of illustrations. The final structure would have to be simple and clear, containing the material essential to teach the crucial concepts of examination and diagnosis.

This book has been written for those who wish to understand more clearly the *clinical* concepts behind neurologic levels. It has been designed to be read sequentially, from cover to cover. Each chapter presents basic neurologic information first, then gives it clinical significance by applying it to the diagnosis of the more common neurologic pathologies. The pattern of teaching thus moves from concept to practice, and from the general rule to its specific application.

However, clinical experience remains the key to real understanding. A book can do no more than present, clearly and concisely, suggested methods of evaluation. In the interest of such clarity, some of the information presented here has been simplified. The clinical findings for each neurologic level have, for example, been stylized to make basic concepts and facts easier to understand; it must be clinical experience that uncovers the variations and exceptions which arise in individual patients. For as Goethe said, "What one knows, one sees."

This book is an expression of my teaching experience at the Albert Einstein College of Medicine, where I have watched orthopaedic, neurosurgical, neurologic, physical medicine, and family practice residents, as well as physical therapists, seek this knowledge. I hope this information, and the special way in which it is organized, provide the understanding necessary to assess the involvement of neurologic levels.

STANLEY HOPPENFELD, M.D.

Acknowledgments

Richard Hutton for his loyalty and devotion to this project. His personal friendship, sense of organization, and knowledge of the English language helped make this book possible. Hugh Thomas for his exceptionally fine art work which illustrates this book. His personal friendship over these years is greatly appreciated.

To my Fellow Attendings at the Albert Einstein College of Medicine, who have been very supportive during the writing and teaching of this material: Uriel Adar, David M. Hirsh, Robert Schultz, Elias Sedlin and Rashmi Sheth. To the British Fellows who have participated in the teaching of Orthopaedic Neurology during their stay with us at "Einstein": Clive Whalley, Robert Jackson, David Gruebel-Lee, David Reynolds, Roger Weeks, Fred Heatley, Peter Johnson, Richard Foster, Kenneth Walker, Maldwyn Griffiths, John Patrick and Robert Johnson. To the Orthopaedic Residents of the Albert Einstein College of Medicine, for allowing me the pleasure of teaching this material.

Hospital for Joint Diseases which awarded me the Frauenthal Fellowship and gave me world exposure to problems of the spine. Rancho Los Amigos Hospital for the education I received in the areas of paraplegia and children's spinal deformities. Lodge Moor Paraplegic Center, where a large amount of my experience in dealing with paraplegic patients was obtained.

Maldwyn Griffith, who took the time to help us reorganize the manuscript, breathing new life into it. John Patrick, for helping me review the manuscript many times, making positive suggestions and helping to prepare a proper bibliography. Al Spiro for taking the time to review the manuscript, making many valuable suggestions, and upholding the special viewpoint of pediatric neurology. Gabriella Molnar in deep appreciation for her review of the initial manuscript, her positive suggestions, and for reviewing the final manuscript. Arthur Abramson in appreciation for his detailed review of the paraplegic and tetraplegic sections. He provided a mature sounding board against which I have tested many ideas. Ed Delagi for reviewing the manuscript and being a friend when one was needed. Charlotte Shelby in appreciation for her review of the manuscript and editorial suggestions during that wonderful Caribbean cruise.

Victor Klig, for all of his help in developing the electronic spinal brace and evaluating neurologic innervation to the paraspinal muscles. Paul Harrington for his brilliance in the surgical approach to the spine and for making me appreciate how to improve spinal alignment, making many patient's lives fuller and richer. W. J. W. Sharrard in appreciation for the time he spent with me during my Fellowship in Sheffield. My knowledge of meningomyelocele children is based on his teaching and most of my understanding of neurologic levels on his basic research of anterior horn cell involvement in patients with poliomyelitis. The late Sir Frank Holdsworth for the time he spent with me discussing spinal problems during my visit to Sheffield. My understanding of spine stability is based upon his work. Mr. Evans and Mr. Hardy of Sheffield in appreciation for their time spent with me at the Paraplegic Center. Jacquelin Perry who, during my Fellowship, spent many hours educating me in the areas of paraplegic and children's deformities. Herman Robbins, who, during my residency, emphasized the neurologic evaluation of patients with spinal problems. Emanuel Kaplan, for opening the door to neurology for orthopaedic surgeons by translating Duchenne's textbook, *Physiology of Motion,* into English and for taking the time to instruct me in these matters. Ben Golub, who has taken the time to evaluate spines and passed this special knowledge on to all of the resident staff. Alex Norman for his special teachings in radiology of the spine. Al Betcher for teaching me neurologic level evaluation of patients with spinal anesthesia. Joe Milgram for all of his help during and after my residency at the Hospital for Joint Diseases.

Alf Nachemson, my long-term friend, with whom I have spent many hours discussing spinal problems. Nathan Allan and Mimi Shore, my personal and professional friends, who have consistently shared their professional and practical knowledge with me. Al Grant and Lynn Nathanson for their help in running the Meningomyelocele Service. To my neurosurgical colleagues, in particular Ken Shulman and Stephen Weitz and Hugh Rosomoff, with whom I have had the pleasure of sharing patient care, surgery, and numerous discussions about neurologic level problems. Roberta and David Ozerkis for a lifetime of frienship and help. Frank Ferrieri, for his friendship and support.

Arthur and Wilda Merker, my friends. Some of the writing of this book was done at their lovely home by the sea. Muriel Chaleff, who through personal efforts, provided a professional touch in preparing this manuscript. Lauretta White who was most devoted in the preparation of this manuscript. Anthea Blamire who was a great help in the typing of this manuscript. Lew Reines for his help in handling the manuscript and production of the book. Fred Zeller in helping to arrange for our book's distribution throughout the world. Brooks Stewart for his help in converting a manuscript and taking it to its final form. To our publishers, J. B. Lippincott Company, who have brought this project to a successful conclusion.

Contents

Introduction.. 1
   Motor Power 1
   Sensation... 1
   Reflex... 2

PART I. NERVE ROOT LESIONS BY NEUROLOGIC LEVEL

   Chapter 1. Evaluation of Nerve Root Lesions Involving the Upper Extremity......... 7
     Testing of Individual Nerve Roots C5 to T1 7
       Neurologic Level C5.................................... 7
       Neurologic Level C6.................................... 13
       Neurologic Level C7.................................... 17
       Neurologic Level C8.................................... 21
       Neurologic Level T1.................................... 23
     Clinical Application 28
       Herniated Cervical Discs................................ 28
       Cervical Neck Sprain versus Herniated Disc 39
       Uncinate Processes and Osteoarthritis...................... 40
       General Tests for Reproducing and Relieving Symptoms of
         Osteoarthritis 42
       Nerve Root Avulsions 42
   Chapter 2. Evaluation of Nerve Root Lesions Involving the Trunk and
     Lower Extremity....................................... 45
     Testing of Individual Nerve Roots T2 to S4 45
       Neurologic Levels T2-T12 45
       Neurologic Levels T12-L3 47
       Neurologic Levels L4 51
       Neurologic Levels L5 57
       Neurologic Levels S1 61
       Neurologic Levels S2, S3, S4........................... 64
     Clinical Application 66
       Herniated Lumbar Discs 66
       Low Back Derangement versus Herniated Disc.............. 67
       Spondylolysis and Spondylolisthesis 68
       Herpes Zoster.. 71
       Poliomyelitis 72

PART II. SPINAL CORD LESIONS BY NEUROLOGIC LEVEL................ 75

   Chapter 3. Cervical Cord Lesions: Tetraplegia.................................... 77
     Evaluation of Individual Cord Levels—C3 to T1 77
       Neurologic Level C3.................................... 77
       Neurologic Level C4.................................... 79

Chapter 3. Cervical Cord Lesions: Tetraplegia — *(Continued)*

Neurologic Level C5... 80
Neurologic Level C6... 81
Neurologic Level C7... 82
Neurologic Level C8... 83
Neurologic Level T1... 83
Upper Motor Neuron Reflex 84
Clinical Application 85
Fractures and Dislocations of the Cervical Spine 85
Herniated Cervical Discs.................................. 91
Tumors of the Cervical Spine............................. 91
Tuberculosis of the Spine................................ 91
Transverse Myelitis 91

Chapter 4. Spinal Cord Lesions Below T1, Including the Cauda Equina 93
Paraplegia 93
Neurologic Level T1-T12.................................. 93
Neurologic Level L1...................................... 94
Neurologic Level L2 94
Neurologic Level L3 94
Neurologic Level L4...................................... 94
Neurologic Level L5...................................... 95
Neurologic Level S1 95
Upper Motor Neuron Reflexes 95
Clinical Application 96
Further Evaluation of Spinal Cord Injuries 96
Herniated Thoracic Discs................................. 100
Evaluation of Spinal Stability to Prevent Further Neurologic
Level Involvement...................................... 101

Chapter 5. Meningomyelocele 107
Determination of Level and Clinical Application 107
Neurologic Level L1/L2 109
Neurologic Level L2/L3 109
Neurologic Level L3/L4 111
Neurologic Level L4/L5 113
Neurologic Level L5/S1 116
Neurologic Level S1/S2 118
Neurologic Level S2/S3 118
Milestones of Development.................................. 118
Unilateral Lesions 119
Hydrocephalus 119
Involvement of the Upper Extremity 119
Suggestions for Examination 120

References 121
Index.. 127

Introduction

The spinal cord is divided into segments. Nerve roots exit the spinal cord at each segmental level, and are numbered in relation to the level from which they exit. There are eight cervical, twelve thoracic, five lumbar, and five sacral nerves. The C5-T1 segments innervate the upper extremity, and the T12-S4 segments the lower extremity; these two sections of the cord have the greatest clinical significance.

Pathology affecting the spinal cord and nerve roots commonly produces symptoms and signs in the extremities according to the specific neurologic levels involved. These levels can usually be diagnosed clinically, since each level of injury has its own characteristic pattern of denervation.

The common denominator in injuries to either the cord or the nerve root lies in the segmental pattern of alteration of motor power, sensation, and reflex in the extremities. Evaluation of the integrity of the neurologic levels depends upon a knowledge of the *dermatomes, myotomes,* and *reflexes.* Different dermatomes (areas of sensation on the skin supplied by a single spinal segment) and myotomes (groups of muscles innervated by a single spinal segment) are affected depending upon the level involved and upon whether the pathology involves the cord or the nerve roots emanating from it. It is through a clinical evaluation of motor power, sensation, and reflex that the correct neurologic level of involvement can be established.

MOTOR POWER

The impulses that supply motor power are transported in the spinal cord via the long tracts, and in particular via the corticospinal tracts. Interruption of the nerve root causes denervation and paralysis of its myotome; interruption of the tract causes spastic paralysis (Fig. I–1). Pressure on the nerve root may produce a decrease in muscle strength that can be evaluated best through the standards set by the National Foundation of Infantile Paralysis, Inc., Committee on After-Effects, and adopted by the American and British Academies of Orthopaedic Surgeons (Table I–1).

In learning to grade a muscle, it is best to remember that a grade 3 muscle can move the joint through a range of motion against gravity. Above grade 3 (grades 4 and 5), resistance is added to the muscle test; below grade 3 (grades 2, 1, and 0), gravity is eliminated as a factor.

Muscle testing should be repeated on a regular basis to determine whether the level of the lesion has changed and created either further muscular paralysis or improvement. Repetitive muscle testing against resistance helps determine whether the muscle fatigues easily, implying weakness and neurologic involvement.

SENSATION

Sensation of pain and temperature is carried in the spinal cord via the lateral spinothalamic

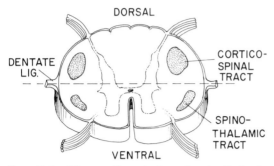

Fɪɢ. I–1. The corticospinal and spinothalamic tracts.

tract, whereas touch is carried in the ventral spinothalamic tract (Fig. I–1). Pathology to the cord or nerve root results in the loss of light touch, followed by loss of sensation of pain. During a recovery from nerve root injury, sensation of pain returns before light touch. The two sensations are tested separately, light touch with a cotton swab, pain with pinpricks.

When testing for pain, use a pin in a gentle sticking motion. The pinpricks should follow in succession, but not too rapidly. A pinwheel is an excellent alternative method of evaluating alterations in sensation, since two neurologic pinwheels can be used simultaneously, one on each side, to permit bilateral comparison. Safety pins may also be used. The use of needles is not recommended since they have cutting surfaces and may injure the patient. Once an area of altered sensation is found, it can be located more precisely by repeated testing from the area of diminished sensation to the area of normal sensation. Sensation tests depend largely upon subjective responses; full cooperation of the patient is necessary.

After sensation is evaluated, the results should be recorded on a dermatome diagram as normal, hyperesthetic (increased), hypesthetic (decreased), dysesthetic (altered), or anesthetic (absent).

REFLEX

The stretch reflex arc is composed of an organ capable of responding to stretch (muscle spindle), a peripheral nerve (axon), the spinal cord synapse, and muscle fibers (Fig. I–2).

TABLE I–1.   MUSCLE GRADING CHART

Muscle Gradations	Description
5 – Normal	Complete range of motion against gravity with full resistance
4 – Good	Complete range of motion against gravity with some resistance
3 – Fair	Complete range of motion against gravity
2 – Poor	Complete range of motion with gravity eliminated
1 – Trace	Evidence of slight contractility. No joint motion
0 – Zero	No evidence of contractility

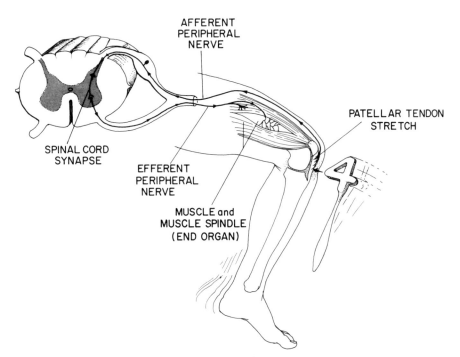

AFFERENT
PERIPHERAL
NERVE

PATELLAR TENDON
STRETCH

SPINAL CORD
SYNAPSE

EFFERENT
PERIPHERAL
NERVE

MUSCLE and
MUSCLE SPINDLE
(END ORGAN)

FIG. I–2. The stretch reflex arc.

Impulses descend from the brain along long (upper motor neuron) tracts to modulate the reflex. As a general rule, an interruption in the basic reflex arc results in the loss of reflex, while pressures on the nerve root itself may decrease its intensity (hyporeflexia). Interruption of the upper motor neuron's regulatory control over the reflex will ultimately cause it to become hyperactive (hyperreflexia).

Reflexes should be reported as normal, increased, or decreased, an evaluation which requires that one side be compared with the other. Bilateral comparison provides a direct, immediately accessible way to detect any alteration in reflexes and is essential for an accurate diagnosis of pathology since the degree of reflex activity varies from person to person.

The concept of determining neurologic levels applies to the evaluation of spinal injuries, developmental anomalies, herniated discs, osteoarthritis, and pathologic processes of the cord itself. All these pathologic processes result in specific segmental distribution of neurologic signs in the extremities because of their direct effect on the spinal cord and nerve roots.

Note that the difference in findings between cord or nerve root pathology as opposed to peripheral nerve injuries is reflected in differences in the distribution of the neurologic findings of motor power, sensation, and reflex. While each dermatome and myotome is innervated at a cord level and by a peripheral nerve, each has its own distinct pattern of innervation.

Part One

Nerve Root Lesions by Neurologic Level

1 Evaluation of Nerve Root Lesions Involving the Upper Extremity

Examination by neurologic level is based upon the fact that the effects of pathology in the cervical spine are frequently manifested in the upper extremity (Fig. 1–1). Problems which affect the spinal cord itself or nerve roots emanating from the cord may surface in the extremity as muscle weakness or abnormality, sensory diminution, and abnormality of reflex; the distribution of neurologic findings depends upon the level involved. Thus, a thorough neurologic testing of the extremity helps determine any involvement of neurologic levels; it may also assist in the evaluation of an assortment of problems originating in the cervical cord or its nerve roots.

The following diagnostic tests demonstrate the relationship between neurologic problems in the upper extremity and pathology involving the cervical nerve roots. For each neurologic level of the cervical spine, motor power, reflexes, and areas of sensation in the upper extremity should be tested so that the level involved can be identified. We have begun individual nerve root testing with C5, the first contribution to the clinically important brachial plexus. Although C1-C4 are not included in our tests because of the difficulty of testing them, it is crucial to remember that the C4 segment is the major innervation to the diaphragm (via the phrenic nerve).

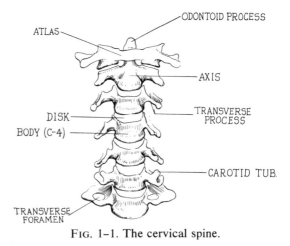

FIG. 1–1. The cervical spine.

TESTING OF INDIVIDUAL NERVE ROOTS: C5 TO T1

Neurologic Level C5

Muscle Testing. The deltoid and the biceps are the two most easily tested muscles with C5 innervation. The deltoid is almost a pure C5 muscle; the biceps is innervated by both C5 and C6, and evaluation of its C5 innervation may be slightly blurred by this overlap.

DELTOID: C5 (AXILLARY NERVE). The deltoid is actually a three-part muscle. The anterior deltoid flexes, the middle deltoid abducts, and the posterior deltoid extends the shoulder;

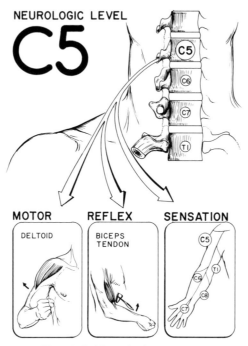

FIG. 1–2. Neurologic level C5.

Shoulder Abduction

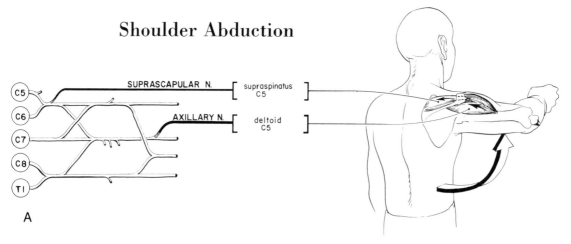

FIG. 1–3A.

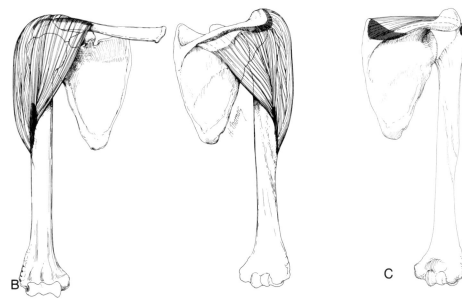

FIG. 1–3B. *Deltoid.*

Origin: Lateral third of clavicle, upper surface of acromion, spine of scapula.

Insertion: Deltoid tuberosity of humerus.

FIG. 1–3C. *Supraspinatus.*

Origin: Supraspinous fossa of scapula.

Insertion: Superior facet of greater tuberosity of humerus, capsule of shoulder joint.

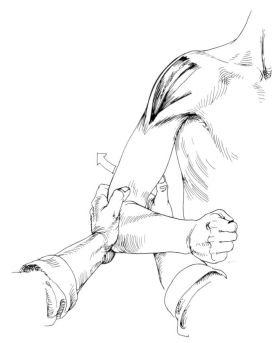

FIG. 1–4. Muscle test for shoulder abduction.

of the three motions, the deltoid acts most powerfully in abduction. Since the deltoid does not work alone in any motion, it may be difficult to isolate it for evaluation. Therefore, note its relative strength in abduction, its strongest plane of motion (Fig. 1–2).

Primary shoulder abductors (Fig. 1–3).
1. Deltoid (middle portion)
   C5, C6 (Axillary nerve)
2. Supraspinatus
   C5, C6 (Suprascapular nerve)
Secondary shoulder abductors
1. Deltoid (anterior and posterior portions)
2. Serratus anterior (by direct stabilizing action on the scapula, since abduction of the shoulder requires a stable scapula).

Stand behind the patient and stabilize the acromion. Slide your stabilizing hand slightly laterally so that, while you stabilize the shoul-

Elbow Flexion and Extension

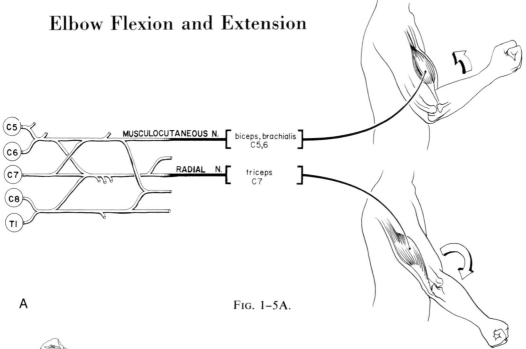

A

FIG. 1–5A.

B   C

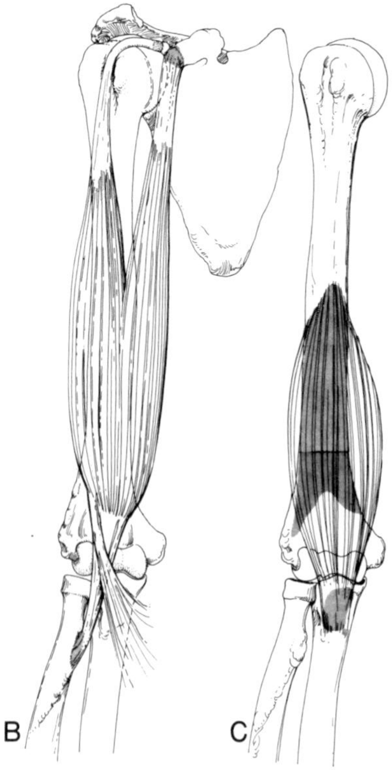

der girdle, you can also palpate the middle portion of the deltoid.

Instruct the patient to abduct his arm with the elbow flexed to 90°. As he moves into abduction, gradually increase your resistance to his motion until you have determined the maximum resistance he can overcome (Fig. 1–4). Record your findings in accordance with the muscle grading chart (see page 2).

FIG. 1–5B. *Biceps Brachii* (left).

Origin: Short head from tip of coracoid process of scapula, long head from supraglenoid tuberosity of scapula.

Insertion: Radial tuberosity and by lacertus fibrosus to origins of forearm flexors.

FIG. 1–5C. *Brachialis* (right).

Origin: Lower two-thirds of the anterior surface of the humerus.

Insertion: Coronoid process and tuberosity of the ulna.

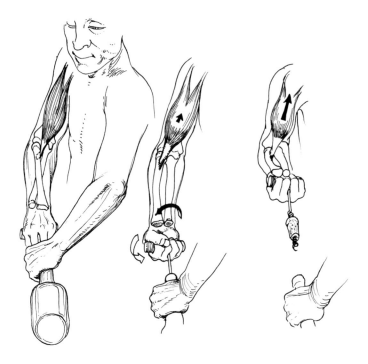

FIG. 1–6. Various functions of the biceps. (Hoppenfeld, S.: Physical Examination of the Spine and Extremities, Appleton-Century-Crofts.)

BICEPS: C5-C6 (MUSCULOCUTANEOUS NERVE). The biceps is a flexor of the shoulder and elbow and a supinator of the forearm (Fig. 1–5); to understand its full function, envision a man driving a corkscrew into a bottle of wine (supination), pulling out the cork (elbow flexion), and drinking the wine (shoulder flexion) (Fig. 1–6).

To determine the neurologic integrity of C5, we shall test the biceps only for elbow flexion. Since the brachialis muscle, the other main flexor of the elbow, is also innervated by C5, testing flexion of the elbow should give a reasonable indication of C5 integrity.

To test flexion of the elbow, stand in front of the patient, slightly toward the side of the elbow being tested. Stabilize his upper extremity just proximal to the elbow joint by cupping your hand around the posterior portion of the elbow. The forearm must remain in supination to prevent muscle substitution that may assist elbow flexion.

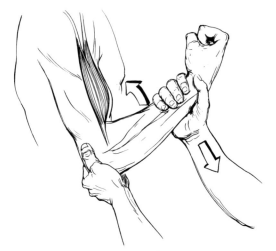

FIG. 1–7. Muscle test for the biceps.

Instruct the patient to flex his arm slowly. Apply resistance as he approaches 45° of flexion; determine the maximum resistance that he can overcome (Fig. 1–7).

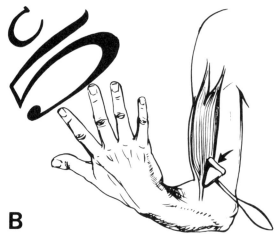

B

Fig. 1–8A. Biceps reflex test.

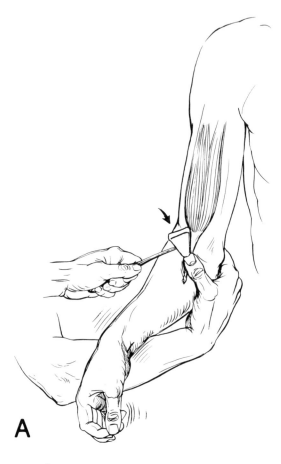

A

Fig. 1–8B. An easy way to remember that the biceps reflex is innervated by C5 is to associate *five* fingers with neurologic level C5.

Reflex Testing

BICEPS REFLEX. The biceps reflex is predominantly an indicator of C5 neurologic integrity; it also has a smaller C6 component. Note that, since the biceps has two major levels of innervation, the strength of the reflex needs only to be slightly weaker than the strength of the opposite side to indicate pathology.

To test the reflex of the biceps muscle, place the patient's arm so that it rests comfortably across your forearm. Your hand should be under the medial side of the elbow, acting as support for the arm. Place your thumb on the biceps tendon in the cubital fossa of the elbow (Fig. 1–8). To find the exact location of the biceps tendon, have the patient flex his elbow slightly. The biceps tendon will stand out under your thumb.

Instruct the patient to relax his extremity completely and to allow it to rest on your forearm, with his elbow flexed to approximately 90°. With the narrow end of a reflex hammer, tap the nail of your thumb. The biceps should jerk slightly, a movement that you should be able to either see or feel. To remember the C5 reflex level more easily, note that when the biceps tendon is tapped, *five* fingers come up in a universal gesture of disdain (Fig. 1–8).

Sensation Testing

LATERAL ARM (AXILLARY NERVE). The C5 neurologic level supplies sensation to the lateral arm, from the summit of the shoulder to the elbow. The purest patch of axillary nerve sensation lies over the lateral portion of the deltoid muscle. This localized sensory area within the C5 dermatome is useful for indicating specific trauma to the axillary nerve as well as general trauma to the C5 nerve root (Fig. 1–9).

Neurologic Level C6

Muscle Testing. Neither the wrist extensor group nor the biceps muscle has pure C6 innervation. The wrist extensor group is innervated partially by C6 and partially by C7; the biceps has both C5 and C6 innervation (Fig. 1–10).

Wrist Extensor Group: C6 (Radial Nerve) (Fig. 1–11)

Radial extensors:

1. Extensor carpi radialis longus and brevis

    Radial Nerve, C6

Ulnar Extensor:

1. Extensor carpi ulnaris, C7

To test wrist extension, stabilize the forearm with your palm on the dorsum of the wrist and your fingers wrapped around it. Then instruct the patient to extend his wrist. When the wrist is in full extension, place the palm of your resisting hand over the dorsum of his hand and try to force the wrist out of the extended position (Fig. 1–12). Normally, you will be unable to move it. Test the opposite side as a means for comparison. Note that the radial wrist extensors, which supply most of the power for extension, are innervated by C6, while the extensor carpi ulnaris is innervated primarily by C7. If C6 innervation is absent and C7 is present, the wrist will deviate to the ulnar side during extension. On the other hand, in a spinal cord injury where C6 is completely spared and C7 is absent, radial deviation will occur.

Biceps: C6 (Musculocutaneous Nerve). The biceps muscle, in addition to its C5 innervation, is partially innervated by C6. Test the biceps by muscle testing flexion of the elbow. (For details, see page 11.)

Reflex Testing

Brachioradialis Reflex. The brachioradialis is innervated by the radial nerve via the C6 neurologic level. To test the reflex, support the patient's arm as you did in testing the biceps reflex. Tap the tendon of the bra-

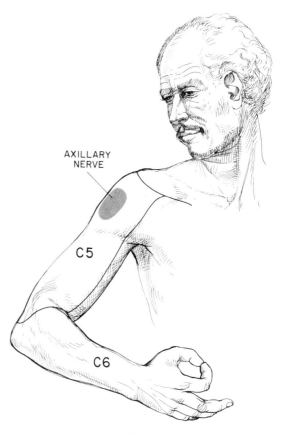

Fig. 1–9. The sensory distribution of the C5 neurologic level.

chioradialis at the distal end of the radius, using the flat edge of your reflex hammer; the tap should elicit a small radial jerk (Fig. 1–13). Test the opposite side, and compare results. The brachioradialis is the preferred reflex for indicating C6 neurologic level integrity.

Biceps Reflex. The biceps reflex may be used as an indicator of C6 neurologic integrity as well as of C5. However, because of this dual innervation, the strength of its reflex need only weaken slightly in comparison to the opposite side to indicate neurologic problems. The biceps reflex is predominantly a C5 reflex.

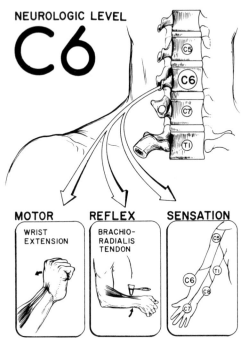

FIG. 1–10. Neurologic level C6.

Wrist Extension and Flexion

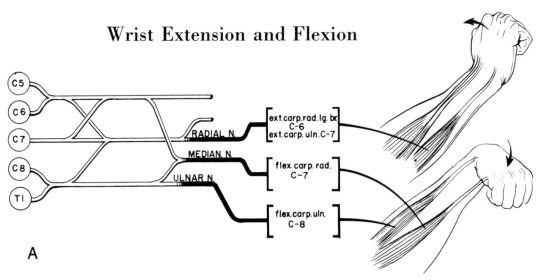

FIG. 1–11A.

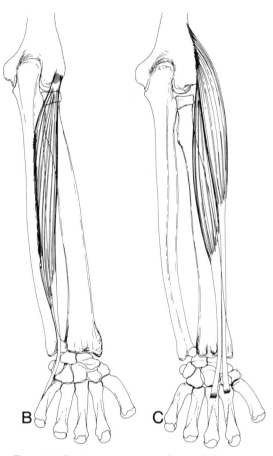

FIG. 1–11B. *Extensor carpi ulnaris* (left).

Origin: From common extensor tendon from lateral epicondyle of humerus, and from posterior border of ulna.

Insertion: Medial side of base of 5th metacarpal bone.

FIG. 1–11C. *Extensor carpi radialis longus* (right).

Origin: Lower third of lateral supracondylar ridge of humerus, lateral intermuscular septum.

Insertion: Dorsal surface of base of 2d metacarpal bone.

FIG. 1–11C. *Extensor carpi radialis brevis* (right).

Origin: From common extensor tendon from lateral epicondyle of humerus, radial collateral ligament of elbow joint, intermuscular septa.

Insertion: Dorsal surface of base of 3d metacarpal bone.

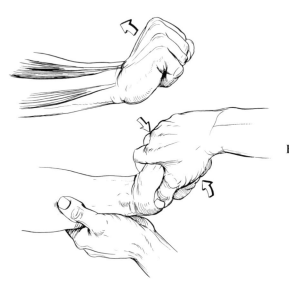

FIG. 1–12. Muscle test for wrist extension.

FIG. 1–13. Brachioradialis reflex test. C-6

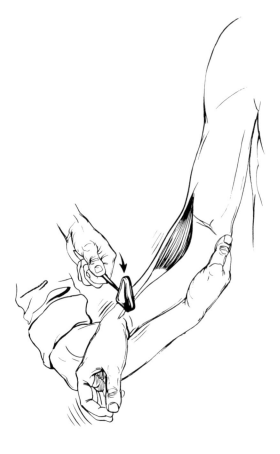

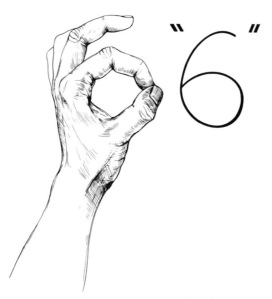

Fig. 1–14. An easy way to remember the sensory distribution of C6.

To test the biceps reflex, tap its tendon as it crosses the elbow. (For details, see page 12.)

Sensation Testing

LATERAL FOREARM (MUSCULOCUTANEOUS NERVE). C6 supplies sensation to the lateral forearm, the thumb, the index finger, and one half of the middle finger. To remember the C6 sensory distribution more easily, form the number six with your thumb, index, and middle fingers by pinching your thumb and index finger together while extending your middle finger (Fig. 1–14).

Neurologic Level C7

Muscle Testing. While the triceps, wrist flexors, and finger extensors are partially innervated by C8, they are predominantly C7 muscles.

TRICEPS: C7 (RADIAL NERVE) (Fig. 1–15). The triceps is the primary elbow extensor. To test it, stabilize the patient's arm just proximal to the elbow and instruct him to extend his arm from a flexed position. Before he reaches 90°, begin to resist his motion until you have discovered the maximum resistance he can overcome (Fig. 1–16). Your resistance should be constant and firm, since a jerky, pushing type of resistance cannot permit an accurate evaluation. Note that gravity is normally a valuable aid in elbow extension; if extension seems very weak, you must account for it, as well as for the weight of the arm. If extension seems weaker than grade 3, test the triceps in a gravity-free plane. Triceps strength is important because it permits the patient to support himself on a cane or standard crutch (Fig. 1–17).

WRIST FLEXOR GROUP: C7 (MEDIAN AND ULNAR NERVES) (Fig. 1–11)

    1. Flexor carpi radialis
        Median nerve, C7
    2. Flexor carpi ulnaris
        Ulnar nerve, C8

(Continued on page 20)

NEUROLOGIC LEVEL
C7

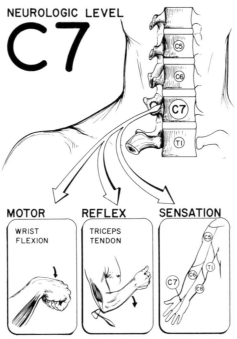

MOTOR	REFLEX	SENSATION
WRIST FLEXION	TRICEPS TENDON	

FIG. 1–15. Neurologic level C7.

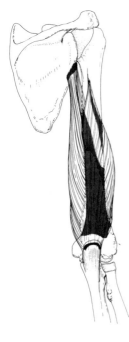

FIG. 1–16A. *Triceps brachii.*

Origin: Long head from infraglenoid tuberosity of scapula, lateral head from posterior and lateral surfaces of humerus, medial head from lower posterior surface of humerus.

Insertion: Upper posterior surface of olecranon and deep fascia of forearm.

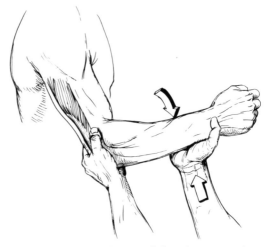

FIG. 1–16B. Muscle test of the triceps muscle.

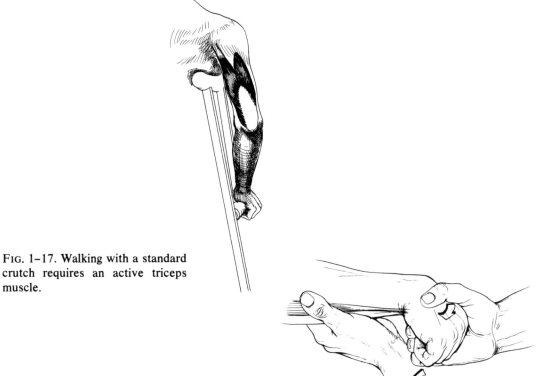

FIG. 1–17. Walking with a standard crutch requires an active triceps muscle.

FIG. 1–18B. Muscle test for the wrist flexors.

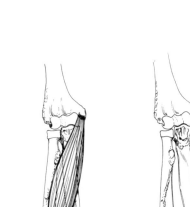

FIG. 1–18A. *Flexor carpi radialis* (left).

Origin: Common flexor tendon from medial epicondyle of humerus, fascia of forearm.

Insertion: Base of 2d and 3d metacarpal bones.

FIG. 1–18A. *Flexor carpi ulnaris* (right).

Origin: Humeral head from common flexor tendon from medial epicondyle of humerus, *ulnar head* from olecranon and dorsal border of ulna.

Insertion: Pisiform, hamate, 5th metacarpal bones.

Finger Extension and Flexion

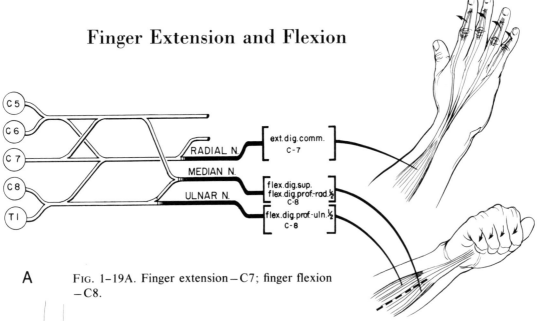

A   FIG. 1–19A. Finger extension — C7; finger flexion — C8.

The flexor carpi radialis (C7) is the more important of these two muscles and provides most of the power for wrist flexion. The flexor carpi ulnaris, which is primarily innervated by C8, provides less power, but acts as an axis for flexion. To understand this, note the ulnar direction that normal flexion takes.

To prepare for the wrist flexion test, instruct the patient to make a fist. The finger flexors can, in some instances, act as wrist flexors; finger flexion removes them as factors during the test, since the muscles have contracted before the test begins. Stabilize the wrist; then instruct the patient to flex his closed fist. When the wrist is in flexion, hold the patient's fingers and try to pull the wrist out of its flexed position (Fig. 1–18).

FIG. 1–19B. *Extensor digitorum.*

Origin: Lateral epicondyle of humerus by common extensor tendon, intermuscular septa.

Insertion: Lateral and dorsal surface of phalanges of medial four digits.

B

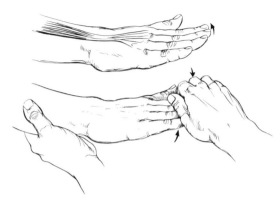

FIG. 1–20. Muscle test for finger extension.

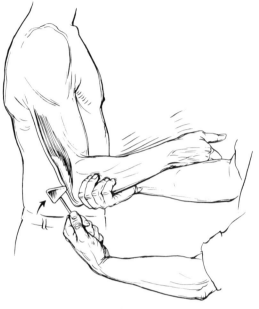

FIG. 1–21. Triceps reflex test.

FINGER EXTENSORS: C7 (RADIAL NERVE) (Fig. 1–19)
1. Extensor digitorum communis
2. Extensor indicis proprius
3. Extensor digiti minimi

To test extension of the fingers, stabilize the wrist in the neutral position. Instruct the patient to extend his metacarpophalangeal joints and flex his interphalangeal joints at the same time. Flexion of the interphalangeal joints prevents the substitution of the intrinsic muscles of the hand for the long finger extensors. Place your hand on the dorsum of the extended proximal phalanges and try to force them into flexion (Fig. 1–20).

Reflex Testing

TRICEPS REFLEX. The triceps reflex is innervated by the C7 component of the radial nerve.

To test the reflex of the triceps muscle, rest the patient's arm on your forearm; the position is exactly the same as it was in the test for the biceps reflex. Instruct the patient to relax his arm completely. When you know that his arm is relaxed (you can feel the lack of tension in the triceps muscle), tap the triceps tendon as it crosses the olecranon fossa (Fig. 1–21). The triceps tendon should jerk slightly, a move-

ment that you can either feel along your supporting forearm or see.

Sensation Testing

MIDDLE FINGER. C7 supplies sensation to the middle finger. Since middle finger sensation is also occasionally supplied by C6 and C8, there is no conclusive way to test C7 sensation.

Neurologic Level C8

Muscle Test.
FINGER FLEXORS (Fig. 1–19)
1. Flexor digitorum superficialis
   Median nerve, C8
2. Flexor digitorum profundis
   Median and ulnar nerves, C8
3. Lumbricals
   Median and ulnar nerves, C8 (T1)

The flexor digitorum profundus, which flexes the distal interphalangeal joint, and the lumbricals, which flex the metacarpo-

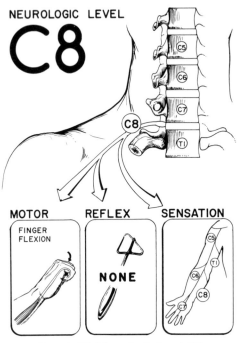

NEUROLOGIC LEVEL

C8

MOTOR | REFLEX | SENSATION

FINGER FLEXION

NONE

FIG. 1–22. Neurologic level C8.

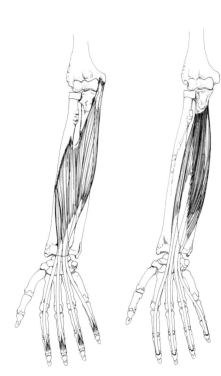

FIG. 1–23A. *Flexor digitorum superficialis* (left).

Origin: Humeral head from common flexor tendon from medial epicondyle of humerus, *ulnar head* from coronoid process of ulna, *radial head* from oblique line of radius.

Insertion: Margins of palmar surface of middle phalanx of medial four digits.

Flexor digitorum profundus (right).

Origin: Medial and anterior surface of ulna, interosseus membrane, deep fascia of forearm.

Insertion: Distal phalanges of medial four digits.

FIG. 1–23B. *Lumbricales.* (See opposite page)

Origin: There are four lumbricales, all arising from tendons of flexor digitorum profundus: 1st from radial side of tendon for index finger, 2d from radial side of tendon for middle finger, 3d from adjacent sides of tendons for middle and ring fingers, 4th from adjacent sides of tendons for ring and little fingers.

Insertion: With tendons of extensor digitorum and interossei into bases of terminal phalanges of medial four digits.

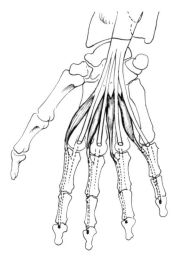

FIG. 1–23B. Lumbricales.

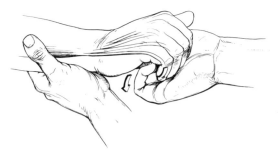

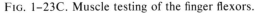

FIG. 1–23C. Muscle testing of the finger flexors.

phalangeal joint, usually receive innervation from the ulnar nerve on the ulnar side of the hand and from the median nerve on the radial side. If there is an injury to the C8 nerve root, the entire flexor digitorum profundus becomes weak, with secondary weakness in all finger flexors. If, however, there is a peripheral injury to the ulnar nerve, weakness will exist only in the ring and little fingers. The flexor digitorum superficialis, which flexes the proximal interphalangeal joint, has only median nerve innervation, and is affected by root injury to C8 and peripheral injuries to the median nerve. (Fig. 1–22).

To test flexion of the fingers, instruct the patient to flex his fingers at all three sets of joints: the metacarpophalangeal joints, the proximal interphalangeal joints, and the distal interphalangeal joints. Then curl or lock your four fingers into his (Fig. 1–23). Try to pull his fingers out of flexion. As you evaluate the results of your test, note which joints fail to hold flexion against your pull. Normally, all joints should remain flexed. To remember the C8 motor level more easily, note that the muscle test has four of your fingers intertwined with four of the patient's; the sum equals 8 (Fig. 1–24).

Sensation Testing

MEDIAL FOREARM (MEDIAL ANTEBRACHIAL CUTANEOUS NERVE). C8 supplies sensation to the ring and little fingers of the hand and the distal half of the forearm. The ulnar side of the little finger is the purest area for sensation of the ulnar nerve (which is predominantly C8), and is the most efficient location for testing. Test the opposite side as a means for comparison, and grade your patient's sensation as normal, diminished (hypoesthesia), increased (hyperesthesia), or absent (anesthesia).

Neurologic Level T1

Test T1 for its motor and sensory components, since T1, like C8, has no identifiable reflex associated with it (Fig. 1–25).

Muscle Testing

FINGER ABDUCTION (Fig. 1–26)
1. Dorsal interossei (D.A.B.)–(The initials indicate that the Dorsal interossei ABduct.)
   Ulnar nerve, T1

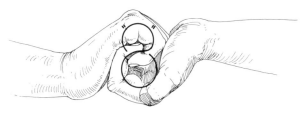

FIG. 1–24. An easy way to remember that C8 innervates the finger flexors.

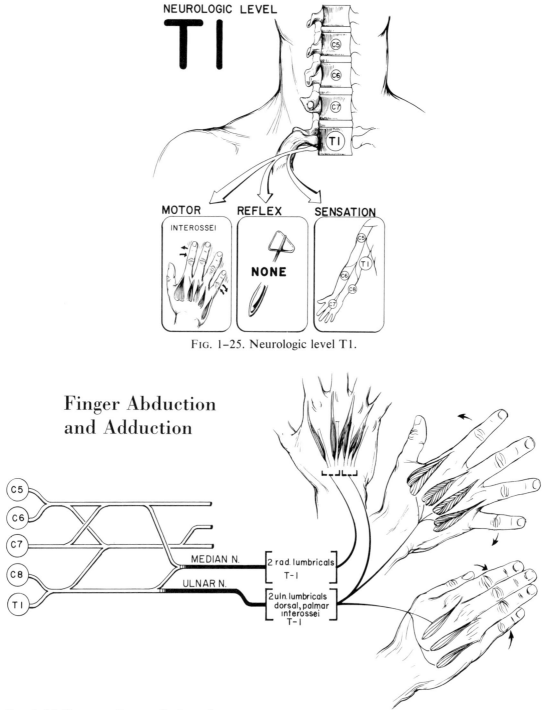

FIG. 1–25. Neurologic level T1.

Finger Abduction and Adduction

FIG. 1–26 (See opposite page for legend)

2. Abductor digiti quinti (fifth finger)
    Ulnar nerve, T1

Note that all small muscles of the hand are innervated by T1. To test finger abduction, instruct the patient to abduct his extended fingers away from the axial midline of the hand. Then pinch each pair of fingers to try to force them together: pinch the index to the middle, ring, and little fingers, the middle to the ring and little fingers, and the ring to the little fingers (Fig. 1–27). Observe any obvious weaknesses between pairs and test the other hand as a means of comparison.

Note that pushing the little finger to the ring finger tests the abductor digiti quinti.

FINGER ADDUCTION (Fig. 1–26)
Primary Adductor
    1. Palmar Interossei (P.A.D.)—(the initials indicate that the Palmar interossei ADduct.)
       Ulnar nerve, C8, T1

To test finger adduction, have the patient try to keep his extended fingers together while you attempt to pull them apart. Test in pairs as follows: the index and middle fingers, the middle and ring fingers, and the ring and little fingers.

Finger adduction can also be checked if you place a piece of paper between two of the patient's extended fingers and pull it out from between. The strength of his grasp should be compared to that of the opposite hand (Fig. 1–28). To remember the T1 neurologic level

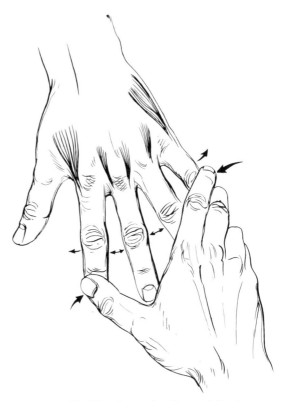

FIG. 1–27. Muscle test for finger abduction.

more easily, pull a *one*-dollar bill from between the extended fingers and associate the *one* dollar with neurologic level *T1*.

Sensation Testing

MEDIAL ARM (MEDIAL BRACHIAL-CUTANEOUS NERVE). T1 supplies sensation to the upper half of the medial forearm and the medial portion of the arm.

Summary

The following is a recommended scheme of testing neurologic levels in the upper extremity. In the neurologic examination of the upper extremity, it is practical to evaluate all motor power first, then all reflexes, and finally sensation. This method permits economy of effort and creates a minimum of disturbance for the patient.

FIG. 1–26. *Interossei dorsales* (page 24).

Origin: There are four dorsal interossei, each arises by two heads from adjacent sides of metacarpal bones.

Insertion: 1st into radial side of proximal phalanx of 2d digit, 2d into radial side of proximal phalanx of 3d digit, 3d into ulnar side of proximal phalanx of 3d digit. 4th into ulnar side of proximal phalanx of 4th digit.

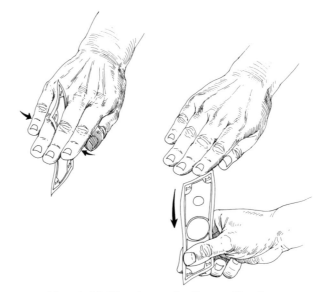

Fig. 1–28. Muscle test for finger adduction.

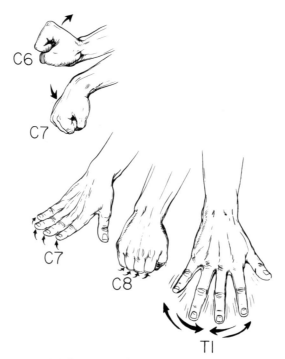

Fig. 1–29. Summary of muscle testing for the upper extremity.

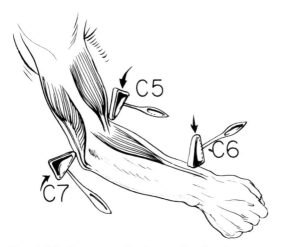

FIG. 1–30. Summary of reflex testing for the upper extremity.

Motor power can be tested almost completely in the wrist and hand with minimal motion and effort for the examiner and patient. Wrist extension (C6), wrist flexion and finger extension (C7), finger flexion (C8), and finger abduction and adduction (T1) can all be performed in one smooth motion. Only C5 must be tested elsewhere, with the deltoid and biceps muscles (Fig. 1–29).

Reflexes can all be obtained in a smooth pattern if the elbow and extremity are stabilized in one position. It is then easy to move the reflex hammer to tap the appropriate tendon — biceps (C5), brachioradialis (C6), and triceps (C7) (Fig. 1–30).

Sensation can also be tested in a smooth pattern. Start proximally on the outer portion of the extremity and move down the extremity (C5, arm; C6, forearm), then across the fingers (C6, C7, C8). Finally, move up the inner border of the extremity (C8, forearm; T1, arm), to the axilla (T2) (Fig. 1–31).

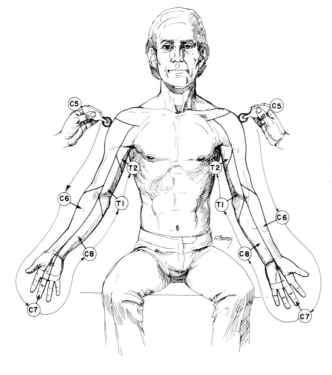

FIG. 1–31. Summary of sensation for the upper extremity.

Neurologic Levels in Upper Extremity

Motor

C5 – Shoulder Abduction
C6 – Wrist extension
C7 – Wrist flexion and finger extension
C8 – Finger flexion
T1 – Finger abduction, adduction

Sensation

C5 – Lateral arm
C6 – Lateral forearm, thumb, and index finger
C7 – Middle finger (variable)
C8 – Medial forearm, ring, and small finger
T1 – Medial arm
T2 – Axilla

Reflex

C5 – Biceps
C6 – Brachioradialis
C7 – Triceps

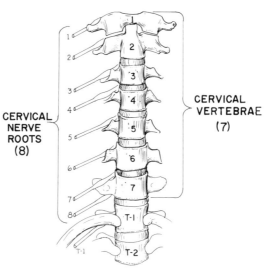

Fig. 1–32. Cervical vertebrae and nerve roots.

CLINICAL APPLICATION OF NEUROLOGIC LEVELS

Herniated Cervical Discs

There are eight cervical nerves and only seven cervical vertebrae; thus, the first cervical nerve exits between the occiput and C1, the sixth between C5 and C6, and the eighth between C7 and T1 (Fig. 1–32). A herniated disc impinges upon the nerve root exiting above the disk and passing through the nearby neural foramen, and results in involvement of one specific neurologic level. For example, a herniated disc between C5 and C6 impinges upon the C6 nerve root (Fig. 1–33).

There is slightly more motion between C5 and C6 than between the other cervical vertebrae (except for between the specialized articulations of the occiput and C1, and C1 and C2) (Fig. 1–34, 1–35). Greater motion causes a greater potential for breakdown, and the incidence of herniated discs and osteoar-

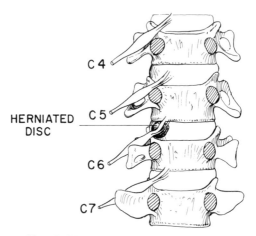

Fig. 1–33. A herniated cervical disc.

thritis is greater at C5-C6 than at any of the other cervical disc spaces. The incidence of herniation increases at C6-C7 as the patient grows older; the reasons for this are not yet known.

To involve the nerve root, the discs must herniate posteriorly. They do so for two reasons: first, the annulus fibrosus is intact and strong anteriorly and defective posteriorly;

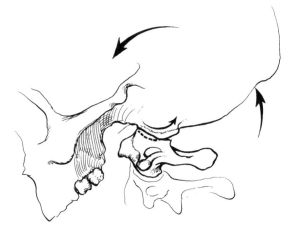

FIG. 1–34. Specialized articulation between the occiput and C1 allowing for 50 per cent of the flexion and extension in the cervical spine.

FIG. 1–35. Specialized articulation between C1 and C2 allowing for 50 per cent of the rotation in the cervical spine.

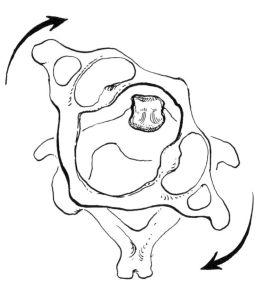

second, the anterior longitudinal ligament is anatomically broader and stronger than the narrower posterior longitudinal ligament. Since a disc usually herniates under pressure, it breaks through in the direction of least resistance, posteriorly. Because of the rhomboidal shape of the posterior longitudinal ligament, the disc also tends to herniate to one side or the other (Fig. 1–36); it is less common to have a midline herniation, since the disc would then have to penetrate the strongest portion of the ligament.

Pain in one arm or the other is symptomatic of herniated cervical discs; the pain usually ra-

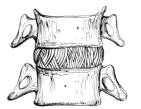

ANT. ANNULUS FIBROSUS

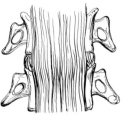

ANT. LONGITUDINAL LIG.

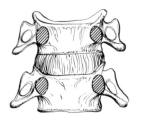

POST. ANNULUS FIBROSUS

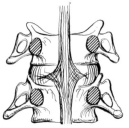

POST. LONGITUDINAL LIG.

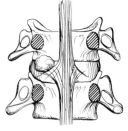

HERNIATED DISC

FIG. 1–36. The anatomic basis for posterior cervical disc herniation.

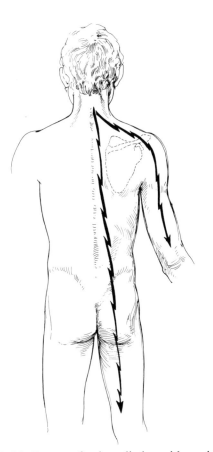

FIG. 1-37. Pattern of pain radiation with a midline herniated cervical disc.

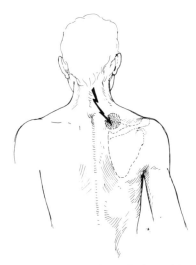

FIG. 1-38. Pattern of pain radiation with a lateral protrusion of a cervical disc.

diates to the hand along the neurologic pathways of the involved root, although, occasionally, the pain may be referred only as far as the shoulder. Coughing, sneezing, or straining usually aggravates the pain and causes it to radiate throughout the involved neurologic distribution in the extremity.

The symptoms and signs caused by a herniated disc vary depending upon the location of the herniation. If the herniation is lateral, as is most common, it may impinge directly upon the nerve root, giving classical root-level neurologic findings. However, if the disc herniates in the midline, the symptoms may be evident in the leg and arm as well (Fig. 1-37).

If the disc protrudes but does not herniate, pain may be referred to the midline of the back in the area of the superior medial portions of the scapulae (Fig. 1-38). Lateral protrusion may send pain along the spinous border of the scapula (most commonly to the superior medial angles), with radiation of pain down the arm, but usually without neurologic findings.

Occasionally, there may be inconsistent findings of neurologic level involvement during the examination. Sometimes the brachial plexus, which usually includes the nerve roots C5 to T1, will begin a level higher (pre-fixed) or a level lower (post-fixed), causing variations in the segmental innervation of the muscles; the findings will reflect this inconsistency in the innervation of the upper extremity. It is also possible that such major inconsistencies are due to brachial plexus or peripheral nerve injuries.

Specific Tests for Locating Herniated Cervical Discs. To establish the exact neurologic level of involvement secondary to a herniated disc, use the neurologic evaluation technique described earlier in the chapter. (Figs. 1-39 to 1-43) (Text continues on page 37.)

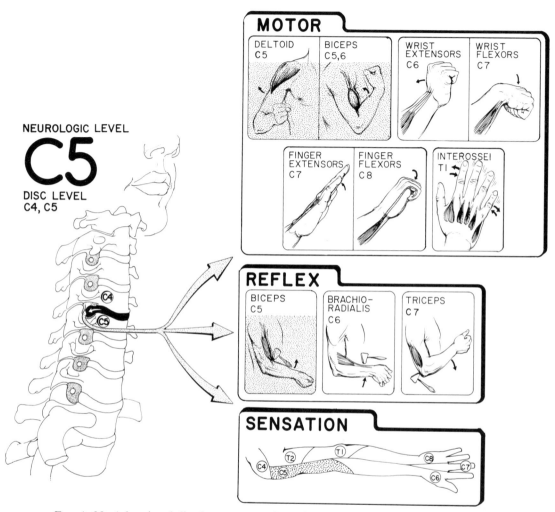

NEUROLOGIC LEVEL
C5
DISC LEVEL
C4, C5

FIG. 1–39. A herniated disc between vertebrae C4 and C5 involves the C5 nerve root.

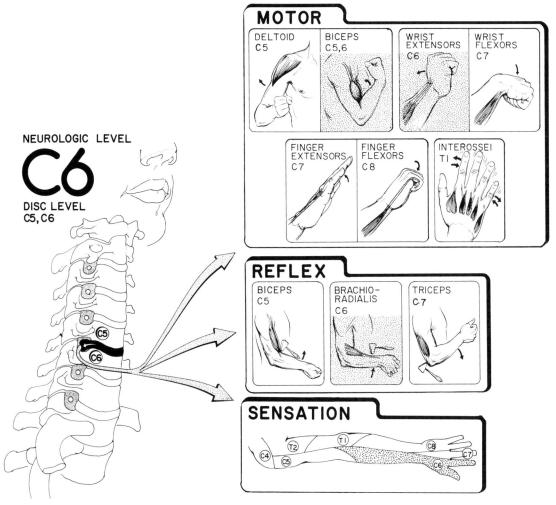

FIG. 1–40. A herniated disc between vertebrae C5 and C6 involves the C6 nerve root. This is the most common level of disc herniation in the cervical spine.

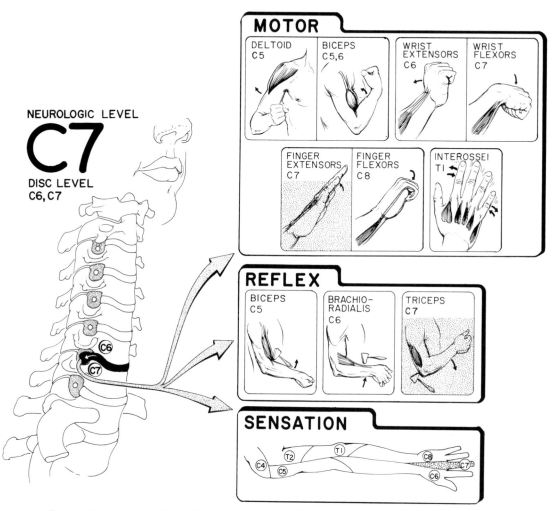

FIG. 1–41. A herniated disc between vertebrae C6 and C7 involves the C7 nerve root.

NEUROLOGIC LEVEL

C8

DISC LEVEL
C7, TI

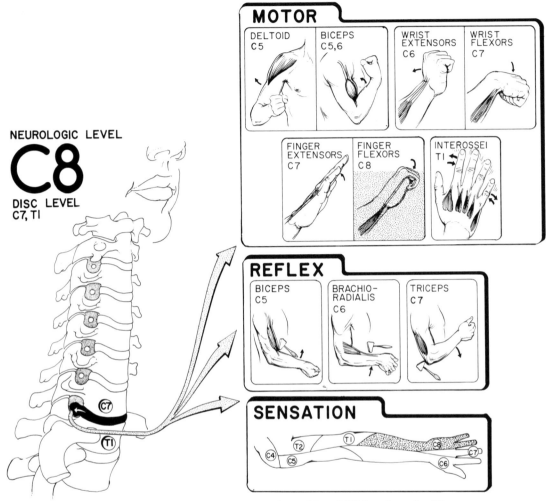

Fig. 1–42. A herniated disc between vertebrae C7 and T1 involves the C8 nerve root.

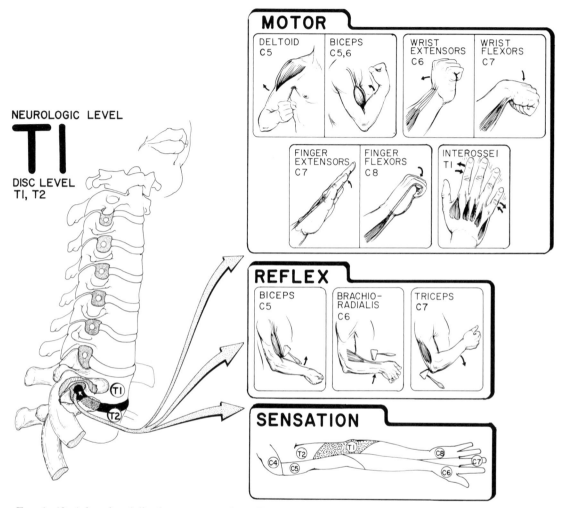

Fig. 1–43. A herniated disc between vertebrae T1 and T2 involves the T1 nerve root. A herniated disc in this area is unusual.

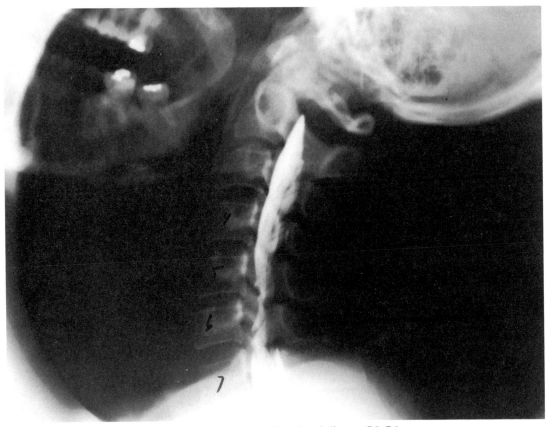

FIG. 1–44. Myelogram: herniated disc at C5-C6.

Table 1–1 summarizes the areas of neurologic level testing. In addition, it demonstrates the clinical application of neurologic level testing to pathology in the cervical spine, especially with regard to the evaluation of herniated discs. Other ways of locating herniated discs are through:

1. The myelogram, which reveals the abnormal protrusion of a herniated disc into the spinal cord, nerve root, or cauda equina at the involved level. It is the most accurate way to detect herniation, but should be reserved and used as a final test. (Fig. 1–44)

2. The electromyogram (EMG), which accurately measures motor potentials. Two weeks after injury to a nerve, abnormal spontaneous electrical discharges appear in the resting muscle (fibrillation potentials and positive sharp waves). These are evidence of a muscle denervation, that can result from herniated discs, nerve root avulsions, or cord lesions. (They can also occur in plexus and peripheral nerve lesions.) It is important that muscles representing each neurologic level (myotome) be sampled for a complete evaluation (see Table 1–1 on next page).

TABLE 1–1. UNDERSTANDING HERNIATED DISCS AND OSTEOARTHRITIS OF THE CERVICAL SPINE

Root	Disc	Muscles	Reflex	Sensation	E. M. G.	Myelogram	Uncinate Process
C5	C4-C5	Deltoid Biceps	Biceps	*Lateral arm* Axillary nerve	Fibrillation or sharp waves in deltoid, biceps †	Bulge in spinal cord C4-C5	C5
C6*	C5-C6	Biceps Wrist extensors	Brachioradialis	*Lateral forearm* Musculocutaneous nerve	Fibrillation or sharp waves in biceps ‡	Bulge in spinal cord C5-C6	C6
C7	C6-C7	Triceps Wrist flexors Finger extensors	Triceps	Middle finger	Fibrillation or sharp waves in triceps §	Bulge in spinal cord C6-C7	C7
C8	C7-T1	Hand intrinsics Finger flexors		*Medial forearm* Med. Ant. Brach. cutaneous nerve	Fibrillation or sharp waves in intrinsic hand muscles ‖	Bulge in spinal cord C7-T1	
T1	T1-T2	Hand intrinsics		*Medial arm* Med. Brach. cutaneous nerve	Fibrillation or sharp waves in hand muscles		

* Most common level of herniation
† Deltoid, rhomboid, supra and infraspinatus muscles
‡ Extensor carpi radialis longus & brevis
§ Triceps, flexor carpi radialis, extensor digitorum longus
‖ Flexor digitorum muscles

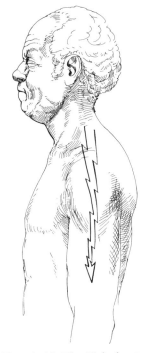

FIG. 1–45. The Valsalva test.

General Test for Herniated Cervical Discs. The Valsalva test is a generalized test which indicates only the presence of a herniated disc. The tests of each neurologic level are more precise and can pinpoint the exact level of involvement.

VALSALVA TEST. The Valsalva test increases the intrathecal pressure. If there is a space-occupying lesion in the cervical canal, such as a herniated disc or a tumor, the patient will develop pain in the cervical spine secondary to the increased pressure. The pain may radiate to the neurologic distribution of the upper extremity that corresponds to the pathologically involved neurologic level.

To perform the Valsalva test, have the patient bear down as if he were moving his bowels while he holds his breath. Then ask him if he feels any increase in pain either in the cervical spine or, by reflection, in the upper extremity (Fig. 1–45). The Valsalva test is a subjective test which requires that the patient answer your questions appropriately; if he is either unable or unwilling to answer, the test is of little value.

Cervical Neck Sprain Versus Herniated Disc

Patients frequently develop neck pain after automobile accidents that cause the cervical spine to whip back and forth (whiplash) or twist (Fig. 1–46A, B). The resulting injury may stretch an individual nerve root, cause a nerve root to impinge upon an osteoarthritic spur, or produce a herniated disc. Patients with neurologic involvement complain of neck pain referred to the medial border of the scapula and radiating down the arm to varying

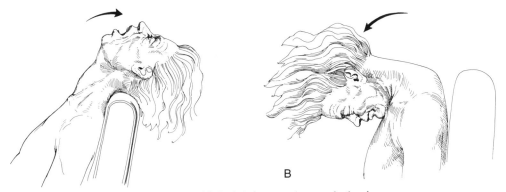

FIG. 1–46A, B. Whiplash injury to the cervical spine.

degrees, as well as of numbness and muscle weakness in the extremity. However, such an injury may simply stretch the posterior or anterior neck muscles, causing a similar neck pain with radiation to the shoulder and medial border of the scapula.

Differentiation between generalized soft tissue injury without neurologic involvement and injury with neurologic involvement can be made by testing the integrity of the neurologic levels innervating the upper extremities. With each patient visit, neurologic testing must be repeated, since an originally quiescent lesion may later clinically manifest itself. Note that the converse is also true: patients who are hospitalized for treatment of neurologic problems may show improved muscle strength, return of a reflex, or return of normal sensation to the involved dermatome.

Many patients continue to complain of cervical pain six months to a year after injury without evidence of either neurologic or ob-jective x-ray findings of pathology. The practitioner should have the confidence, despite patient pressure, to continue conservative (nonoperative) therapy, knowing that the patient may have a permanent soft tissue injury not involving the anterior primary nerve roots or the intervertebral cervical discs.

The Uncinate Processes and Osteoarthritis

The uncinate processes are two ridges of bone which originate on the superior lateral surface of the cervical vertebrae. They help to stabilize the individual vertebra, and participate in the formation of the neural foramen (Fig. 1–47). Enlargements or osteoarthritis involving the uncinate process may encroach upon the neural foramen and directly compress the exiting nerve root or limit the amount of room in which it can move (Fig. 1–48).

The neural foramen and the portion of the uncinate process encroaching upon it can be

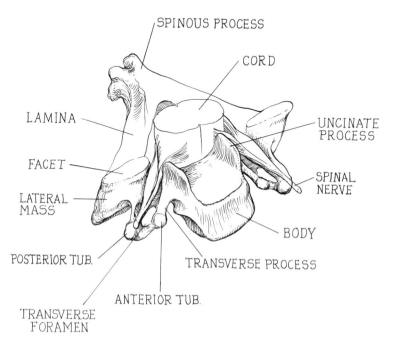

FIG. 1–47. The anatomy of a cervical vertebra.

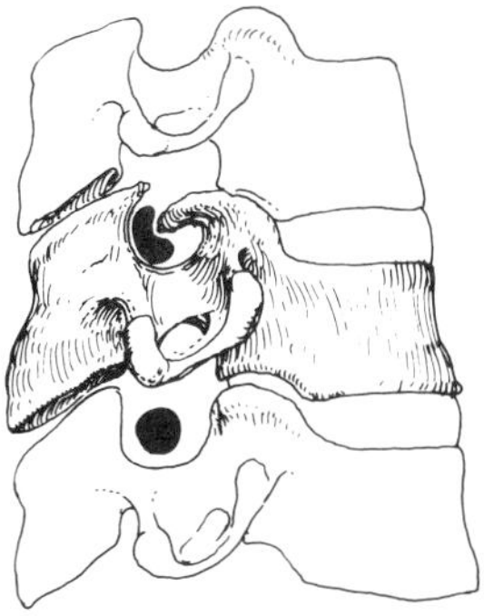

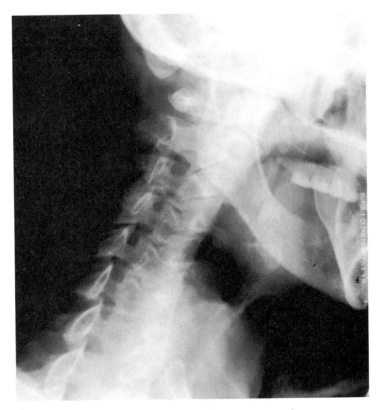

FIG. 1–48. Osteoarthritis of the uncinate process.

seen best on an oblique roentgenogram (Fig. 1–49). Note that the nerve roots emerge at a 45° angle from the cord and vertebral body, the same angle that exists between the neural foramen and the vertebral body. An osteophyte from the uncinate process has little clinical significance unless it is accompanied by symptoms. Clinical problems may arise after an automobile accident, when a patient with a narrowed neural foramen may place excessive strain on the nerve root lying in it because of the extreme extension/flexion of the head and neck and the subsequent reactive

FIG. 1–49. Narrowed neural foramen secondary to osteoarthritis of the uncinate process. C3-C4

edema of the nerve root. Note that the narrowed foramen frequently has the roentgenographic appearance of a figure eight, a configuration which does not allow room for the posttraumatic swelling of the nerve and results in pain. Pain and neurologic findings are naturally found in the involved neural distribution in the upper extremity. For example, trauma affecting the C6 nerve root may result in decreased sensation to the lateral forearm, muscle weakness to the wrist extensors, and an absent brachioradialis reflex (Fig. 1–35). It is also possible, however, that the only symptom is referred pain to the superior medial angle and medial border of the scapula.

Where there is more motion, there is more chance of breakdown, and uncinate process enlargement secondary to osteoarthritis is most often found at the C5-C6 bony level.

General Tests for Reproducing and Relieving Symptoms of Osteoarthritis

Distraction Test. The cervical spine distraction test gives an indication of the effect of neck traction in relieving pain. Distraction relieves pain caused by the narrowing of the neural foramen (leading to nerve root compression) by widening the foramen, as well as by relieving pressure on the joint capsules around the facet joints; it may also help relieve muscle spasm by relaxing the contracted muscles involved.

To perform the cervical spine distraction test, place the open palm of one hand under the patient's chin and the other hand on his occiput. Gradually lift (distract) his head so that the neck is relieved of its weight (Fig. 1–50). Determine whether he experiences any relief from pain.

Compression Test. The cervical spine compression test determines whether the patient's pain is increased when the cervical spine is compressed. Pain caused by narrowing of the neural foramen, pressure on the facet joints, or muscle spasm may be increased by compres-

sion. The compression test may also faithfully reproduce pain referred down the upper extremity from the cervical spine; in doing so, it may assist in locating the neurologic level of existing pathology.

To perform the compression test, press upon the top of the patient's head while he is either sitting or lying down; discover whether there is any corresponding increase in pain either in the cervical spine or down the extremity. Note the exact distribution of this pain and whether it follows any previously described dermatome (Fig. 1–51).

Nerve Root Avulsions

Cervical nerve roots are frequently avulsed from the cord during motorcycle accidents. When a rider is thrown from his cycle, his head and neck are forced laterally and his shoulder is depressed by the impact with the ground, causing the cervical nerve roots to stretch and finally avulse (Fig. 1–52). The C5 and C6 nerve roots are the roots most commonly avulsed.

Physical examination shows the obvious results: with the loss of the C5 root, there is total motor paralysis among the C5 myotome and sensory deficit along the C5 dermatome. The deltoid muscle is paralyzed, sensation along the upper lateral portion of the arm is hypesthetic or anesthetic, and the biceps reflex (C5-C6) is diminished or absent. The myelogram shows a visable sacculation of dye at the point of the avulsion, the origin of the C5 nerve root between the C4 and C5 vertebrae. Such a lesion is not amenable to surgical repair. The injury is permanent; no recovery is to be expected.

Although C5 and C6 are the most commonly avulsed roots, the C8 and T1 may also be avulsed. If the cyclist strikes the ground with his shoulder hyperabducted, the lowest roots of the brachial plexus are usually the ones injured, while the C5 and C6 nerve roots remain intact.

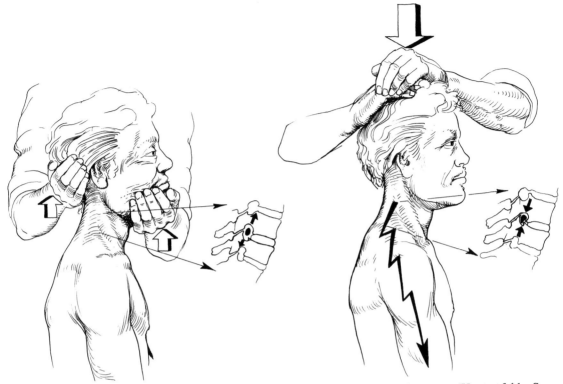

FIG. 1–50. Distraction test (Hoppenfeld, S.: Physical Examination of the Spine and Extremities, Appleton-Century-Crofts).

FIG. 1–51. Compression test (Hoppenfeld, S.: Physical Examination of the Spine and Extremities, Appleton-Century-Crofts).

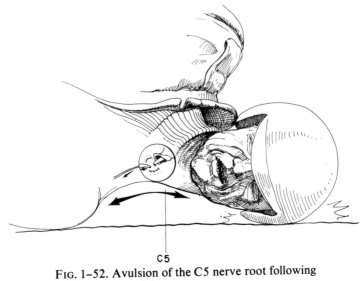

C5

FIG. 1–52. Avulsion of the C5 nerve root following a motorcycle accident.

2 Evaluation of Nerve Root Lesions Involving the Trunk and Lower Extremity

Manifestations of pathology involving the spinal cord and cauda equina, such as herniated discs, tumors, or avulsed nerve roots, are frequently found in the lower extremity. Understanding the clinical relationship between various muscles, reflexes, and sensory areas in the lower extremity and their neurologic levels (cord levels) is particularly helpful in detecting and locating spinal problems with greater accuracy and ease.

To make the relationship between the spine and the lower extremity clear, the neurologic examination of the lumbar spine will be divided into tests of each neurologic level and its dermatomes and myotomes. Thus, for each neurologic level of the lower spinal cord, the muscles, reflexes, and sensory areas which most clearly receive innervation from it will be tested.

TESTING OF INDIVIDUAL NERVE ROOTS, T2 TO S4

Neurologic Levels T2 to T12

Muscle Testing

INTERCOSTALS. The intercostal muscles are segmentally innervated and are difficult to evaluate individually.

RECTUS ABDOMINUS. The rectus abdominus muscles are segmentally innervated by the primary anterior divisions of T5 to T12 (L1), with the umbilicus the dividing point between T10 and T11.

Beevor's sign (Fig. 2–1) tests the integrity of the segmental innervation of the rectus abdominus muscles. Ask the patient to do a quarter sit-up with his arms crossed on his chest. While he is doing this, observe the umbilicus. Normally, it should not move at all when the maneuver is performed. If, however, the umbilicus is drawn up or down or to one side or the other, be alerted to possible asymmetrical involvement of the anterior abdominal muscles.

Sensory Testing. Sensory areas for each nerve root are shown in Figure 4–1. The sensory area for T4 crosses the nipple line, T7 the xiphoid process, T10 the umbilicus, and T12 the groin. There is sufficient overlap of these areas for no anesthesia to exist if only one nerve root is involved. However, hypoesthesia is probably present.

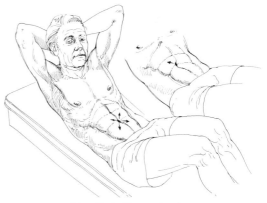

FIG. 2–1. Beevor's sign.

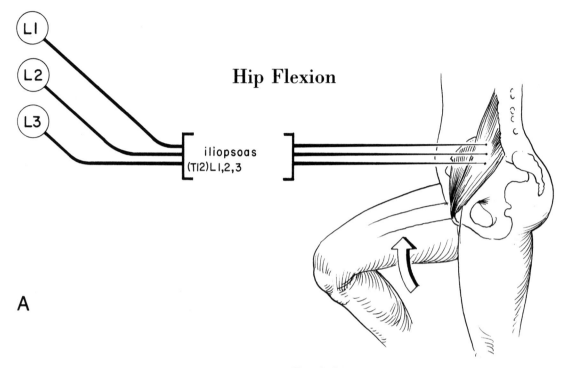

Hip Flexion

A

Fɪɢ. 2–2A. (T12), L1, 2, 3 – Hip flexion.

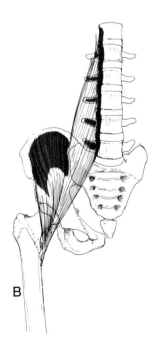

B

Fɪɢ. 2–2B. *Iliopsoas.*

Origin: Anterior surface of the bodies of all lumbar vertebrae and their transverse processes and corresponding intervertebral discs. Upper two thirds of the iliac fossa.

Insertion: Lesser trochanter of femur.

Neurologic Levels T12-L3

Muscle Testing. There is no specific muscle test for each root. The muscles that are usually tested are the iliopsoas (T12, L1, L2, L3), the quadriceps (L2, L3, L4) and the adductor group (L2, L3, L4).

ILIOPSOAS: (BRANCHES FROM [T12], L1, L2, L3) (Fig. 2–2). The iliopsoas muscle is the main flexor of the hip. To test it, instruct the patient to sit on the edge of the examining table with his legs dangling. Stabilize his pelvis by placing your hand over his iliac crest and have him actively raise his thigh off the table. Now place your other hand over the distal femoral portion of his knee and ask him to raise his thigh further as you resist (Fig. 2–3). Determine the maximum resistance he can overcome. Then repeat the test for the opposite iliopsoas muscle and compare muscle strengths. Since the iliopsoas receives innervation from several levels, a muscle which is only slightly weaker than its counterpart may indicate neurologic problems.

In addition to possible neurologic pathology, the iliopsoas may become weak as a result of an abscess within its substance; the patient may then complain of pain during muscle testing. The muscle may also become weak as a result of knee or hip surgery.

QUADRICEPS: ˎL2, L3, L4 (FEMORAL NERVE) (Fig. 2–4). To test the quadriceps functionally, instruct the patient to stand from a squatting position. Note carefully whether he stands straight, with his knees in full extension, or whether he uses one leg more than the other. The arc of motion from flexion to extension should be smooth. Occasionally, the patient may only be able to extend the knee smoothly until the last 10°, finishing the mo-

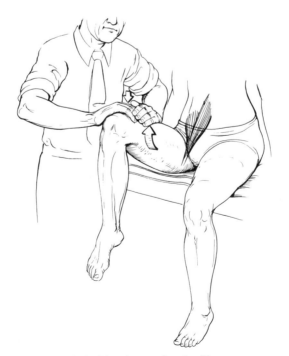

FIG. 2–3. Muscle test for the iliopsoas.

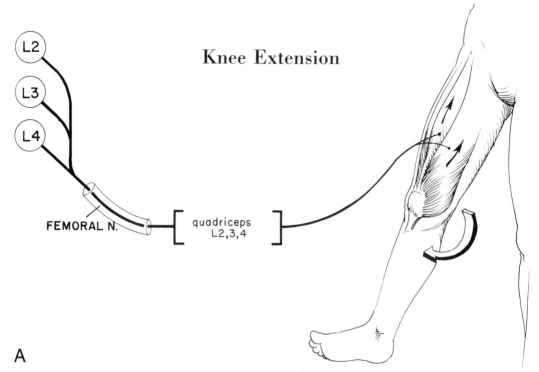

Knee Extension

FEMORAL N.

[quadriceps
L2,3,4]

A

FIG. 2–4A. L2, 3, 4 – Knee extension.

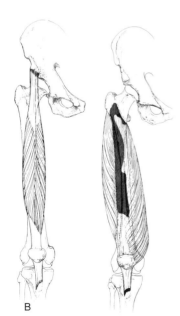

B

FIG. 2–4B. *Rectus femoris.*

Origin: Rectus femoris is a "two joint" muscle that has two heads of origin. Straight head: from anterior inferior iliac spine. Reflected head: from groove just above brim of acetabulum.

Insertion: Upper border of patella, and then into the tibial tubercle via the infrapatellar tendon.

FIG. 2–4C.
Vastus intermedius.

Origin: Upper two-thirds of anterior and lateral surface of femur.

Insertion: Upper border of the patella with the rectus femoris tendon and then, via the infrapatellar tendon into tibial tubercle.

Vastus lateralis.

Origin: Capsule of hip joint, intertrochanteric line, gluteal tuberosity, linea aspera.

Insertion: Proximal and lateral border of patella, and into tibial tubercle via the infrapatellar tendon.

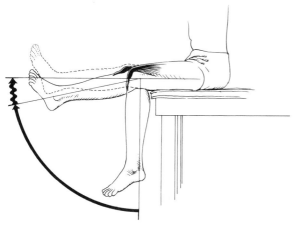

FIG. 2–5. Extension lag. (Hoppenfeld, S.: Physical Examination of the Spine and Extremities, Appleton-Century-Crofts).

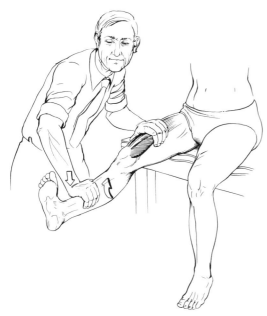

FIG. 2–6. Muscle test for the quadriceps.

Vastus Medialis

Origin: Lower half of intertrochanteric line, linea aspera, medial supracondylar line, medial intermuscular septum, tendon of adductor magnus.

Insertion: Medial border of patella and into tibial tubercle via the infrapatellar tendon.

tion haltingly and with great effort. This faltering in the last 10° of extension is called *extension lag*; it occurs because the last 10°-15° of knee extension requires at least 50 percent more muscle power than the rest (according to Jacqueline Perry). Extension lag is frequently seen in association with quadriceps weakness. Sometimes, the patient may be unable to extend his knee through the last 10° with even the greatest effort (Fig. 2–5).

To test the quadriceps manually, stabilize the thigh by placing one hand just above the knee. Instruct the patient to extend his knee as you offer resistance just above the ankle joint. Palpate the quadriceps during the test with your stabilizing hand (Fig. 2–6). Note that the quadriceps weakness can also be due to a reflex decrease in muscle strength following knee surgery or to tears within the substance of the muscle itself.

HIP ADDUCTOR GROUP: L2, L3, L4 (OBTURATOR NERVE) (Fig. 2–7). Like the quadriceps, the hip adductors can be tested as a massive grouping. Have the patient lie supine or on his side and instruct him to abduct his legs. Place your hand on the medial sides of both knees and have him adduct his legs against your resistance (Fig. 2–8). Determine the maximum resistance he can overcome.

Reflexes. Although the patellar tendon reflex is supplied by L2, L3, and L4, it is predominantly L4 and will be tested as such.

Sensory Testing. Nerves from L1, L2, and L3 provide sensation over the general area of the anterior thigh between the inguinal ligament and the knee. The L1 dermatome is an oblique band on the upper anterior portion of the thigh, immediately below the inguinal ligament. The L3 dermatome is an oblique band on the anterior thigh, immediately above the kneecap. Between these two bands, on the anterior aspect of the midthigh, lies the L2 dermatome (Fig. 2–9).

Sensory testing, with its bands of individual dermatomes, is a more accurate way of eva-

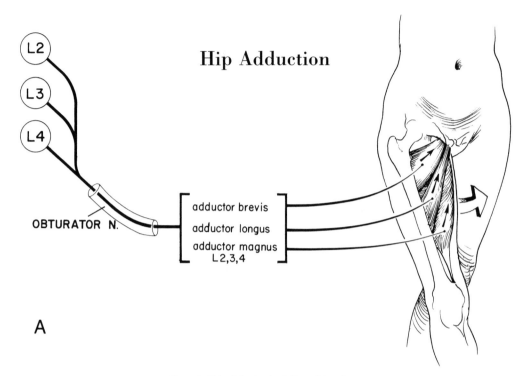

FIG. 2–7A. L2, 3, 4 – Hip adduction.

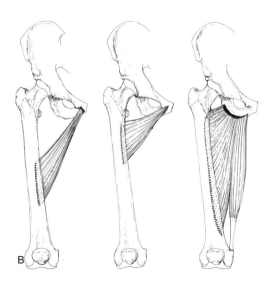

FIG. 2–7B. *Adductor brevis* (center).
   Origin: Outer surface of inferior ramus of pubis.
   Insertion: Line extending from lesser trochanter to linea aspera and upper part of linea aspera.

Adductor longus (left).
   Origin: Anterior surface of the pubis in the angle between crest and pubic symphysis.
   Insertion: Linea aspera, middle half of medial lip.

Adductor magnus (right).
   Origin: Ischial tuberosity, inferior rami of ischium and pubis.
   Insertion: Line extending from greater trochanter to linea aspera. The entire length of linea aspera, medial supracondylar line, and adductor tubercle of the femur.

luating neurologic levels T12, L1, L2, and L3 than motor testing, which lacks individual representative muscles. There are also no representative reflexes for these levels, making it even more difficult to diagnose an exact neurologic level. Neurologic levels L4, L5, and S1 are represented by individual muscles, dermatomes, and reflexes, and are easier to diagnose.

Neurologic Level L4

Muscle Testing

TIBIALIS ANTERIOR: L4 (DEEP PERONEAL NERVE) (Fig. 2–11). The tibialis anterior muscle is predominantly innervated by the L4 segmental level; it also receives L5 innervation. To test the muscle in function, ask the patient to walk on his heels with his feet inverted. The tendon of the tibialis anterior muscle becomes visible as it crosses the anteromedial portion of the ankle joint and is quite prominent as it proceeds distally towards its insertion. Pa-

tients with weak tibialis anterior muscles are unable to perform this functional dorsiflexion-inversion test; they may also exhibit "drop foot," or steppage gait.

To test the tibialis anterior manually, instruct the patient to sit on the edge of the examining table. Support his lower leg, and place your thumb in a position that makes him dorsiflex and invert his foot to reach it. Try to force the foot into plantar flexion and eversion by pushing against the head and shaft of the first metatarsal; palpate the tibialis anterior muscle as you test it (Fig. 2–12).

Reflex Testing

PATELLAR TENDON REFLEX. The patellar tendon reflex is a deep tendon reflex, mediated through nerves emanating from the L2, L3,

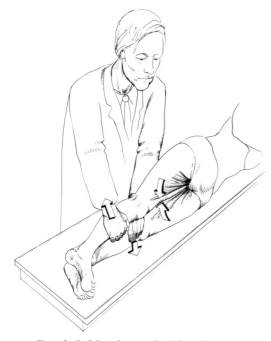

FIG. 2–8. Muscle test for hip adductors.

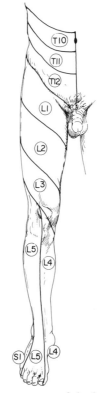

FIG. 2–9. Dermatomes of the lower extremity.

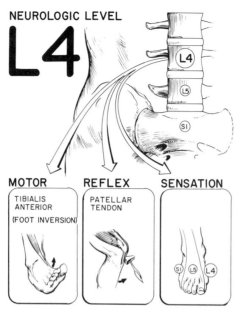

NEUROLOGIC LEVEL

FIG. 2–10. Neurologic level L4.

Foot Inversion

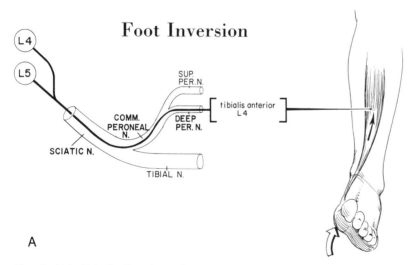

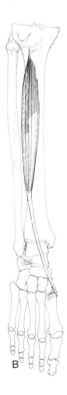

A

FIG. 2–11A. L4, 5 – Foot inversion.

FIG. 2–11B. *Tibialis anterior.*
   Origin: Lateral condyle of tibia, upper two-thirds of the anterolateral surface of tibia, interosseus membrane.
   Insertion: Medial and plantar surfaces of medial cuneiform bone, base of 1st metatarsal bone.

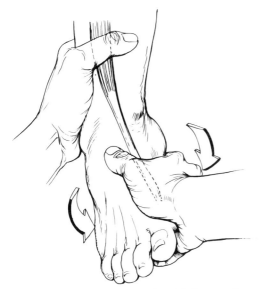

FIG. 2–12. Muscle test for the tibialis anterior.

and L4 nerve roots (predominantly from L4). For clinical application, the patellar tendon reflex should be considered an L4 reflex; however, because it receives innervation from L2 and L3 as well as from L4, the reflex will still be present, although significantly weakened, even if the L4 nerve root is completely severed. The reflex is almost never totally absent. However, in primary muscle, nerve root, or anterior horn cell disease, the reflex can be totally absent.

To test the patellar tendon reflex, ask the patient to sit on the edge of the examining table with his legs dangling. (He may also sit on a chair with one leg crossed over his knee or, if he is in bed, with his knee supported in a few degrees of flexion) (Fig. 2–13). In these positions, the infrapatellar tendon is stretched and primed. Palpate the soft tissue depression on either side of the tendon in order to locate it accurately, and attempt to elicit the reflex by tapping the tendon at the level of the knee joint with a short, smart wrist action. If the reflex is difficult to obtain, reinforce it by having the patient clasp his hands

(continued on p. 56)

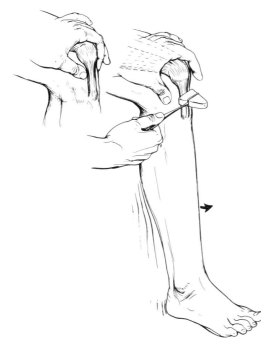

FIG. 2–13. Patellar tendon reflex.

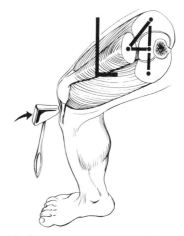

FIG. 2–14. An easy way to remember that the patellar tendon reflex is innervated by L4 is to associate the *four* quadriceps muscles with the neurologic level *L4*.

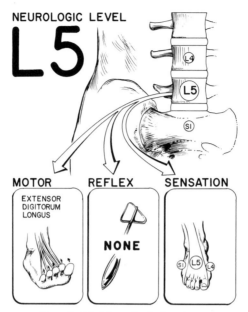

FIG. 2–15. Neurologic level L5.

Foot Dorsiflexion
(Ankle Extension)

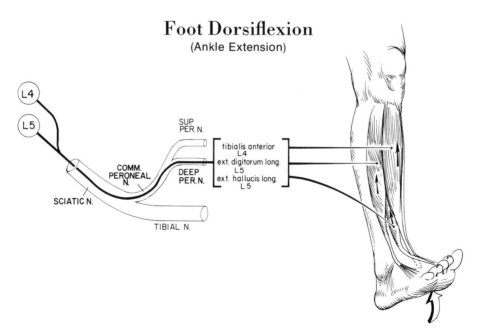

FIG. 2–16. L4, 5 – Foot dorsiflexion (ankle extension).

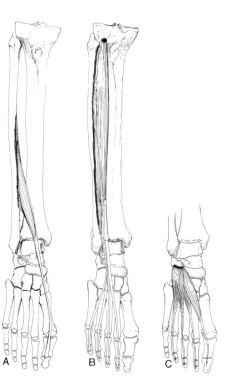

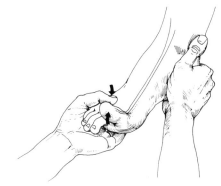

FIG. 2–18A. Muscle test of the extensor hallucis longus muscle.

FIG. 2–17A. *Extensor hallucis longus.*

Origin: Middle half of anterior surface of fibula, adjacent interosseous membrane.

Insertion: Dorsal surface of base of distal phalanx of great toe.

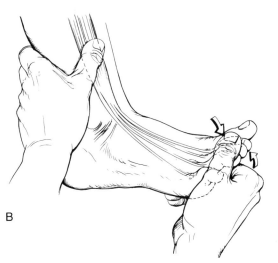

B

FIG. 2–17B. *Extensor digitorum longus.*

Origin: Upper three-fourths of anterior surface of fibula, interosseous membrane.

Insertion: Dorsal surface of middle and distal phalanges of lateral four toes.

FIG. 2–18B. Muscle test for toe extensors.

FIG. 2–17C. *Extensor digitorum brevis.*

Origin: Forepart of upper and lateral surface of calcaneus, sinus tarsi.

Insertion: First tendon into dorsal surface of base of proximal phalanx of great toe, remaining three tendons into lateral sides of tendons of extensor digitorum longus.

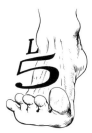

C

FIG. 2–18C. An easy way to remember that the toe extensors are innervated by neurologic level L5.

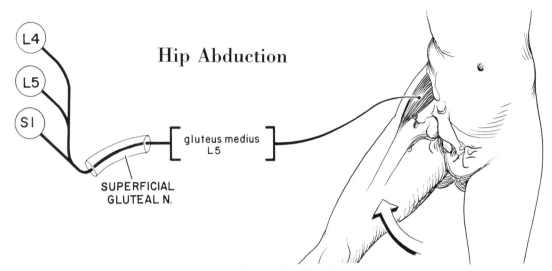

FIG. 2–19. L4, 5, S1 — Hip abduction.

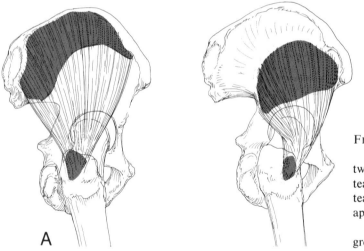

FIG. 2–20A. *Gluteu*
Origin: Outer surfa
tween iliac crest and
teal line above to th
teal line below, as we
aponeurosis.
Insertion: Later
greater trochanter.

and attempt to pull them apart as you tap the tendon. Repeat the procedure on the opposite leg, and grade the reflex as normal, increased, decreased, or absent. To remember the neurologic level of the reflex, associate the fact that *four* muscles constitute the quadriceps muscle with the L*4* of the patellar tendon reflex (Fig. 2–14).

The reflex may be affected by problems other than neurologic pathology. F
if the quadriceps has been traumati
patient has undergone recent surgery
knee, or if there is knee joint effusion
reflex may be absent or diminished.

Sensory Testing. The L4 dermatome covers the medial side of the leg and extends to the medial side of the foot. The knee joint is the dividing line between the L3 dermatome above and the L4 dermatome below. On the leg, the sharp crest of the tibia is the dividing line between the L4 dermatome on the medial side and the L5 dermatome on the lateral side.

Neurologic Level L5

Muscle Testing (Fig. 2–15, 2–16)
1. Extensor hallucis longus
2. Extensor digitorum longus and brevis
3. Gluteus medius

EXTENSOR HALLUCIS LONGUS: L5, (DEEP BRANCH OF THE PERONEAL NERVE). The tendon of the extensor hallucis longus passes in front of the ankle joint lateral to the tibialis anterior. Test it functionally by having the patient walk on his heel, with his foot neither inverted nor everted. The tendon should stand out clearly on the way to its insertion at the proximal end of the distal phalanx of the great toe. To test the extensor hallucis longus manually, have the patient sit on the edge of the ⸍ble. Support the foot with one hand around ⸍caneus and place your thumb in such a position that he must dorsiflex his great toe to reach it. Oppose this dorsiflexion by placing your thumb on the nail bed of the great toe and your fingers on the ball of the foot; then pull down on the toe (Fig. 2–17). If your thumb crosses the interphalangeal joint, you will be testing the extensor hallucis brevis as well as the longus; make certain that you apply resistance distal to the interphalangeal joint so that you are testing only the extensor hallucis longus. Note that a fracture of the great toe or other recent trauma will produce apparent muscle weakness in the extensor hallucis longus.

EXTENSOR DIGITORUM LONGUS AND BREVIS: L5, (DEEP PERONEAL NERVE). Test the extensor digitorum longus in function by instructing the patient to walk on his heels, as he did for the extensor hallucis longus. The tendon of the extensor digitorum longus should stand out on the dorsum of the foot, crossing in front of the ankle mortise and fanning out to insert by slips into the dorsal sur-

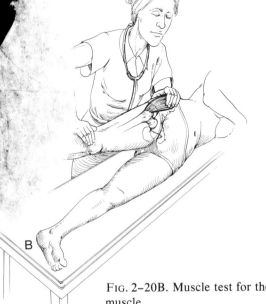

FIG. 2–20B. Muscle test for the gluteus medius muscle.

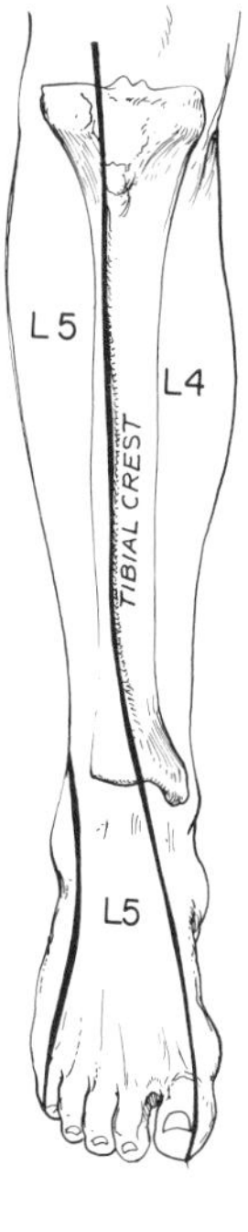

FIG. 2–21. L5 sensory dermatome.

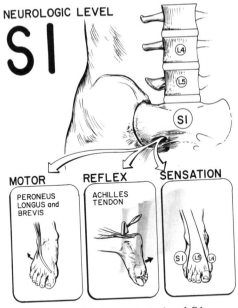

FIG. 2–22. Neurologic level S1.

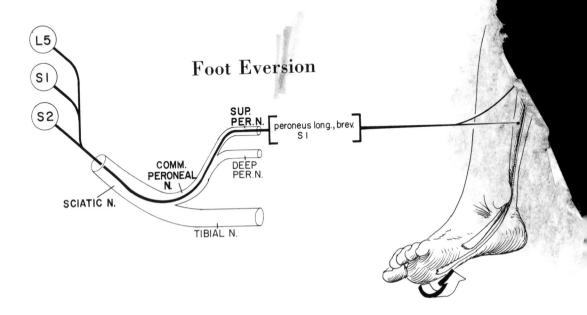

FIG. 2–23. S1—Foot eversion.

faces of the middle and distal phalanges of the lateral four toes.

For the manual test, the patient may remain seated on the edge of the table. Secure the ankle with one hand around the calcaneus and place the thumb of your free hand in such a position that he must extend his toes to reach it. Oppose this motion by pressing on the dorsum of the toes and attempting to bend them plantarward (Fig. 2–18). They should be virtually unyielding.

GLUTEUS MEDIUS: L5, (SUPERIOR GLU-TEAL NERVE) (Fig. 2–19). To test the gluteus medius, have the patient lie on his side. Stabilize his pelvis with one hand and instruct him to abduct his leg. Allow the leg to abduct fully before you resist by pushing against the lateral thigh at the level of the knee joint (Fig. 2–20). To prevent the muscle substitution that may take place if the hip is allowed to flex, make sure it remains in a neutral position throughout the test.

Reflex Testing. There is no easily elicited reflex supplied by the L5 neurologic level. Although the tibialis posterior muscle provides an L5 reflex, it is difficult to elicit routinely. If, after you have performed sensory and motor tests, you are not certain of the integrity of the L5 level, you should try to elicit the *tibialis posterior reflex* by holding the forefoot in a few degrees of eversion and dorsiflexion, and by tapping the tendon of the tibialis posterior muscle on the medial side of the foot just before it inserts into the navicular tuberosity. Normally, you should elicit a slight plantar inversion response.

Sensory Testing. The L5 dermatome covers the lateral leg and dorsum of the foot. The crest of the tibia divides L5 from L4. To make the distinction between L4 and L5 clearer, palpate the crest of the tibia from the knee distally as it angles toward the medial malleolus. All that is lateral to the crest, including the dorsum of the foot, receives sensory innervation from L5 (Fig. 2–21).

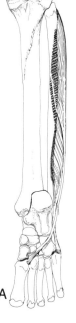

FIG. 2–24A. *Peroneus longus.*

Origin: Head and proximal two-thirds of lateral surface of fibula.

Insertion: Lateral side of medial cuneiform bone, base of 1st metatarsal bone.

Peroneus brevis.

Origin: Distal two-thirds of lateral surface of fibula, adjacent intermuscular septa.

Insertion: Styloid process of base of 5th metatarsal bone.

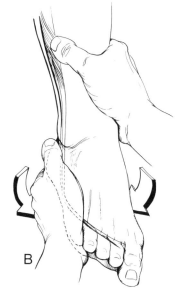

FIG. 2–24B. Muscle test for the peronei muscles.

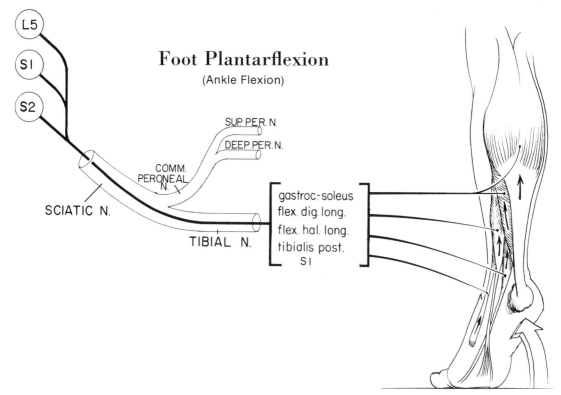

Foot Plantarflexion
(Ankle Flexion)

L5

S1

S2

SUP. PER. N.

DEEP PER. N.

COMM. PERONEAL N.

SCIATIC N.

TIBIAL N.

gastroc-soleus
flex. dig. long.
flex. hal. long.
tibialis post.
S1

Fig. 2–25. L5, S1, 2 — Foot plantarflexion (ankle flexion).

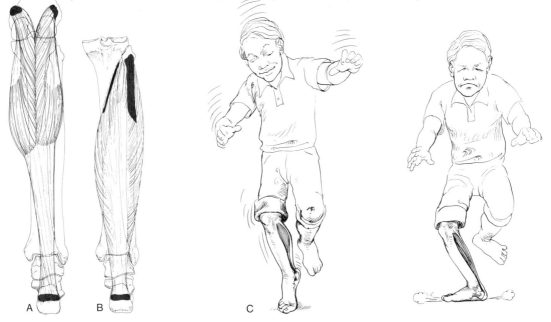

A   B   C

Neurologic Level S1

Muscle Testing

1. Peroneus longus and brevis
2. Gastrocnemius-soleus muscles
3. Gluteus maximus

PERONEUS LONGUS AND BREVIS: S1, (SUPERFICIAL PERONEAL NERVE) (Fig. 2–23). The peronei may be tested together in function. Since they are evertors of the ankle and foot, ask the patient to walk on the medial borders of his feet. The peronei tendons should become prominent just before they turn around the lateral malleolus, pass on either side of the peroneal tubercle (the brevis above, the longus below), and run to their respective insertions.

To test the peronei muscles manually, have the patient sit on the edge of the table. Secure the ankle by stabilizing the calcaneus and place your other hand in a position that forces him to plantarflex and evert his foot to reach it with his small toe. Oppose this plantarflexion and eversion by pushing against the head and shaft of the fifth metatarsal bone with the palm of your hand (Fig. 2–24); avoid applying pressure to the toes, since they may move.

FIG. 2–26A. *Gastrocnemius.*

Origin: Medial head: from medial condyle and adjacent part of femur. Lateral head: from lateral condyle and adjacent part of femur.

Insertion: Into posterior surface of calcaneus by calcaneal tendon (Achilles tendon).

FIG. 2–26B. *Soleus.*

Origin: Posterior surface of head and upper third of the fibula, popliteal and middle third of medial border of tibia, tendinous arch between tibia and fibula.

Insertion: Into posterior surface calcaneus by calcaneal tendon.

FIG. 2–26C. Muscle test for the gastrocnemius-soleus muscle group.

GASTROCNEMIUS-SOLEUS MUSCLES: S1, S2, (TIBIAL NERVE) (Fig. 2–25). Since the gastrocnemius-soleus group is far stronger than the combined muscles of your arm and forearm, it is difficult to detect small amounts of existing weakness; the group is thus a poor choice for manual muscle testing and should be observed in function. Ask the patient to walk on his toes; he will be unable to do so if there is gross muscle weakness. If the test is normal, instruct him to jump up and down on the balls of his feet, one at a time, forcing the calf muscles to support almost two and a half times the body's weight. If he lands flat-footed or is otherwise incapable of performing this test, there is weakness in the calf muscle (Fig. 2–26). Obviously, elderly people or patients with back pain cannot be expected to perform this portion of the functional test. Ask these patients to stand on one leg and rise up on their toes 5 times in succession. Inability to complete this test indicates calf muscle weakness.

GLUTEUS MAXIMUS: S1, (INFERIOR GLUTEAL NERVE) (Fig. 2–27). To test the gluteus maximus functionally, have the patient stand from a sitting position without using his hands. To test it more accurately for strength, ask him to lie prone on the examining table with his hips flexed over the edge and his legs dangling. Have him bend his knee to relax the hamstring muscles so that they cannot assist the gluteus maximus in hip extension. Place your forearm over his iliac crest to stabilize the pelvis, leaving your hand free to palpate the gluteus maximus muscle. Then ask him to extend his hip. Offer resistance to hip extension by pushing down on the posterior aspect of his thigh just above the knee joint; as you perform the test, palpate the gluteus maximus muscle for tone (Fig. 2–28).

Reflex Testing

ACHILLES TENDON REFLEX. The Achilles tendon reflex is a deep tendon reflex, mediated through the triceps surae. It is supplied pre

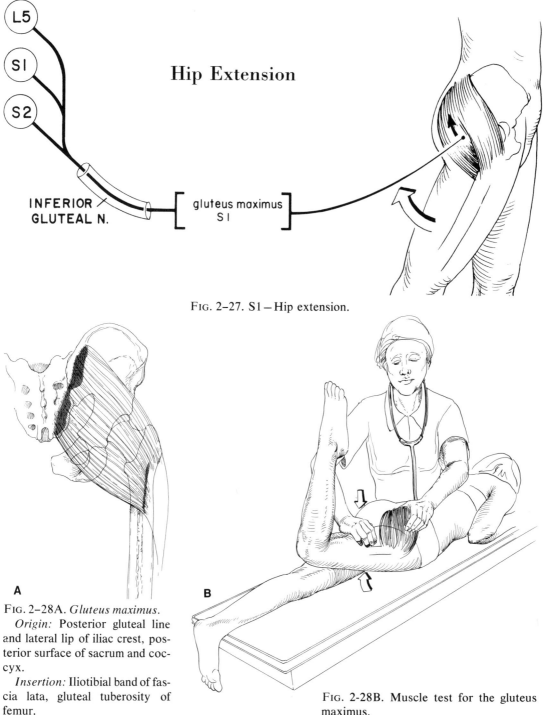

Hip Extension

INFERIOR
GLUTEAL N.

gluteus maximus
S I

FIG. 2–27. S1 – Hip extension.

A

FIG. 2–28A. *Gluteus maximus.*

Origin: Posterior gluteal line and lateral lip of iliac crest, posterior surface of sacrum and coccyx.

Insertion: Iliotibial band of fascia lata, gluteal tuberosity of femur.

B

FIG. 2-28B. Muscle test for the gluteus maximus.

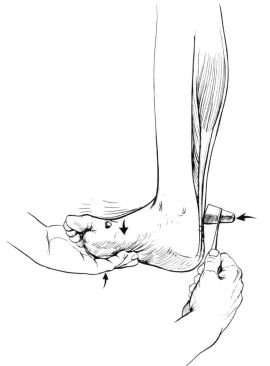

FIG. 2–29. Test of the tendon of Achilles reflex.

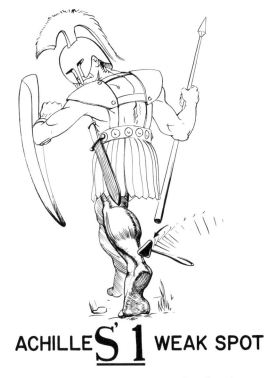

ACHILLES' 1 WEAK SPOT

FIG. 2-30. An easy way to remember that the tendon of Achilles reflex is an S1 reflex.

dominantly by nerves emanating from the S1 cord level. If the S1 root is cut, the Achilles tendon reflex will be virtually absent.

To test the Achilles tendon reflex, ask the patient to sit on the edge of an examining table with his legs dangling. Put the tendon into slight stretch by gently dorsiflexing the foot. Place your thumb and fingers into the soft tissue depressions on either side to locate the Achilles tenson accurately, and strike it with the flat end of a neurologic hammer to induce a sudden, involuntary plantar flexion of the foot (Fig. 2–29). It may be helpful to reinforce the reflex by having the patient clasp his hands and try to pull them apart (or push them together) just as the tendon is being struck. To remember the S1 reflex more easily, associate "AchilleS' 1 weak spot" with the reflex. (Fig. 2-30).

There are various alternate methods of testing the Achilles tendon reflex, some of which are described below. Choose the appropriate method, depending upon the condition of the particular patient that you are examining.

If the patient is bedridden, cross one leg over his opposite knee so that movement of the ankle joint is unhindered. Prime the tendon by slightly dorsiflexing the foot with one hand on the ball of the foot and strike the tendon. If he is lying prone in bed, ask him to flex his knee to 90° and prime the tendon by slightly dorsiflexing his foot before performing the test. If his ankle joint is swollen, or if it is prohibitively painful to tap the Achilles tendon directly, have him lie prone with his ankle over the edge of the bed or examining table. Press the forepart of your fingers against the ball of his foot to dorsiflex it and strike your

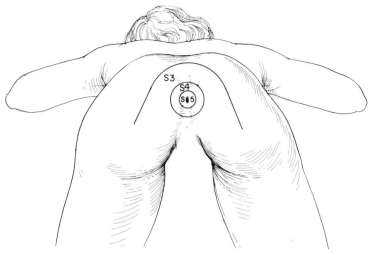

Fig. 2–31. Sensory dermatomes S2, 3, 4, 5.

fingers with the neurologic hammer. A positive reflex is present if the gastrocnemius muscle contracts and the foot plantar flexes slightly. You should be able to detect this motion through your hand.

Sensory Testing. The S1 dermatome covers the lateral side and a portion of the plantar surface of the foot (Fig. 2–9).

Neurologic Levels S2, S3, S4

Nerves emanating from the S2 and S3 neurologic levels supply the intrinsic muscles of the foot. Although there is no efficient way to isolate these muscles for testing, you should inspect the toes for clawing, possibly caused by denervation of the intrinsics. S2, S3, and S4 are also the principal motor supply to the bladder, and neurologic problems which affect the foot may affect it as well.

Reflex Testing. Note that there is no deep reflex supplied by S2, S3, and S4. There is, however, a *superficial anal reflex.* To test it, touch the perianal skin; the anal sphincter muscle (S2, S3, S4) should contract (wink) in response.

Sensory Testing. The dermatomes around the anus are arranged in three concentric rings, receiving innervation from S2 (outermost ring), S3 (middle ring), and S4-S5 (innermost ring) (Fig. 2–31).

Summary

The following is a suggested clinical scheme for most neurologic level testing in the lower extremity. It is practical to evaluate all motor power first, then all sensation, and finally all reflexes.

Most **muscle testing** of the involved lower extremity can be performed with a minimum of effort and motion for examiner and patient if it is generally confined to the foot. Muscle test across the foot from the medial to the lateral side; the tibialis anterior on the medial side of the foot is innervated by L4, the extensor digitorum longus and brevis on the top of the foot by L5, and the peronei on the lateral side of the foot by S1.

Sensation can also be tested in a smooth, continuous pattern across the dorsum of the foot from medial to lateral. The medial border of the foot receives innervation from L4, the top of the foot from L5, and the lateral border

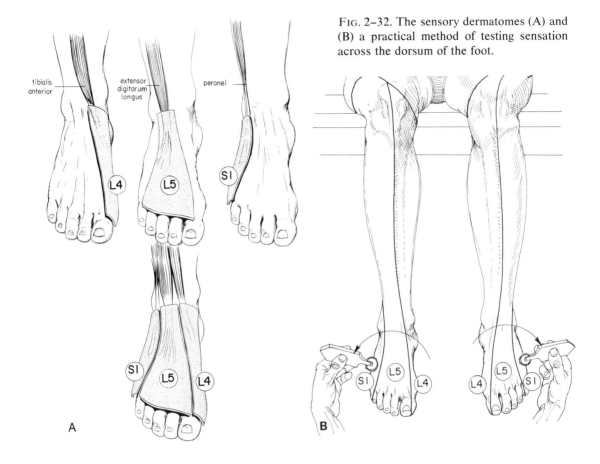

FIG. 2–32. The sensory dermatomes (A) and (B) a practical method of testing sensation across the dorsum of the foot.

of the foot from S1 (Fig. 2–32). It is practical to test sensation in each extremity simultaneously to obtain instant comparison. The skin over a muscle is usually innervated by the same neurologic level as the muscle it covers.

Reflexes can be tested smoothly as well. With the patient seated, the appropriate tendons—infrapatellar tendon, L4; tendon of Achilles, S 1—are easily tested.

NEUROLOGIC LEVELS IN LOWER EXTREMITY

Motor
- L3 – Quadriceps (L2, L3, L4)
- L4 – Tibialis anterior
- L5 – Toe extensors
- S1 – Peronei

Sensation
- T12 – Lower abdomen just proximal to inguinal ligament
- L1 – Upper thigh just distal to inguinal ligament
- L2 – Mid thigh
- L3 – Lower thigh
- L4 – Medial leg—medial side of foot
- L5 – Lateral leg—dorsum of foot
- S1 – Lateral side of foot
- S2 – Longitudinal strip, posterior thigh

Reflex
- L4 – Patellar
- L5 – Tibalis posterior (difficult to obtain)
- S1 – Achilles tendon

TABLE 2–1. UNDERSTANDING HERNIATED LUMBAR DISCS

Root	Disc	Muscles	Reflex	Sensation	E.M.G.	Myelogram
L4	L3-L4	Tibialis anterior	Patellar	Medial leg	Fibrillation or sharp waves in tibialis anterior	Bulge in spinal cord adjacent to L3-L4
L5	L4-L5	Extensor hallucis longus	None (Tibialis posterior)	Lateral leg and dorsum of foot	Fibrillation or sharp waves in extensor hallucis longus†	Bulge in spinal cord adjacent to disc L4-L5
S1	L5-S1*	Peroneus longus & brevis	Achilles tendon	Lateral foot	Fibrillation or sharp waves in peroneus longus & brevis‡	Bulge in spinal cord adjacent to disc L5-S1

* Most common level of herniation
† Extensor digitorum longus and brevis, medial hamstring, gluteus medius muscles
‡ Flexor hallucis longus, gastrocnemius, lateral hamstring, gluteus maximus muscles

CLINICAL APPLICATION OF NEUROLOGIC LEVELS

Herniated Lumbar Discs

Lumbar discs, like cervical discs, usually herniate posteriorly rather than anteriorly and to one side rather than in the midline; the anatomic reasons for each type of herniation are the same (see page 28), and the disc usually impinges only upon one of the two nerve roots at each level (Fig. 2–33). The patient usually complains of pain radiating into one leg or the other, and rarely of pain radiating into both legs at the same time.

Note that there is a special relationship between the nerve roots of the cauda equina and the disc space. Before it exits through the neural foramen, the nerve root turns at approximately a 45° angle around the pedicle of its vertebra. Because the pedicle is situated in the upper third of the vertebral body, the nerve root, which is relatively tethered to it, never crosses the disc space below and thus is usually not involved in any herniations of the disc within that space (Fig. 2–34). A nerve root is commonly involved only in herniations of the disc located *above* its point of exit. For example, the L5 nerve root crosses the disc space between L4 and L5, then turns around the pedicle of L5, and leaves the spinal canal via the neural foramen before it reaches the L5-S1 disc space. It may be affected by an L4-L5 herniation, but not by one between L5 and S1. Thus, a patient whose symptoms are manifested along the L5 distribution has a potential herniation in the disc space *above* the L5 vertebra.

The L4-L5 and L5-S1 articulations have the greatest motion in the lumbar spine. Greater motion causes an increased potential for breakdown, and the incidence of herniated discs is greater at L4-L5 and L5-S1 than at any other lumbar disc space in the entire spine.

Table 2–1 delineates the applicable tests for the most clinically relevant neurologic levels.

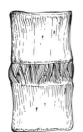

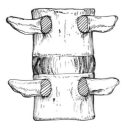

ANT. ANNULUS FIBROSUS   ANT. LONGITUDINAL LIG.

POST. ANNULUS FIBROSUS   POST. LONGITUDINAL LIG.

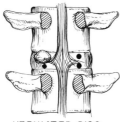

HERNIATED DISC

FIG. 2–33. The anatomic basis for posterior lumbar disc herniation.

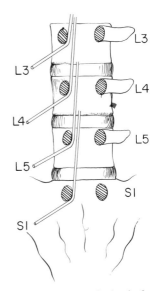

FIG. 2–34. The anatomic basis for nerve root impingement by a herniated disc.

It applies most critically to problems of herniated discs (Fig. 2–35, 2–36, 2–37, 2–38).

Although this table reflects precise neurologic levels, the clinical picture may not be as clear. The reasons for discrepancies are numerous. For example, a nerve root may occasionally carry elements of adjacent nerve roots. Thus, the L4 root may contain components of L3 or L5. In addition, a single disc herniation may involve two nerve roots. This applies particularly to the L4-L5 disc, which may compress not only L5 root but also the S1 root, particularly if the herniation is in the midline. Disc herniation occasionally occurs at more than one level, giving an atypical neurologic pattern.

Low Back Derangement versus Herniated Disc

Patients frequently develop "low back" pain after lifting heavy objects or falling, or after a violent automobile accident which throws or twists them around the interior of the car. These patients complain of back pain (point tenderness or pain across the lower lumbar spine) with radiation to varying degrees around the posterior superior iliac spines and down the back of the leg.

Complaints of a generalized backache or low back derangement without neurologic involvement can be differentiated from those with neurologic involvement by testing the neurologic levels innervating the lower extremity. The tests should be repeated with each visit, since a loss of function not apparent in the initial examination, a further loss of muscle strength, reflex, or sensation in the involved neurologic level, or an improvement from the initial findings (as a result, perhaps, of treatment) may occur.

Unless there is evidence either of an alteration in reflex, sensation, or motor power or of

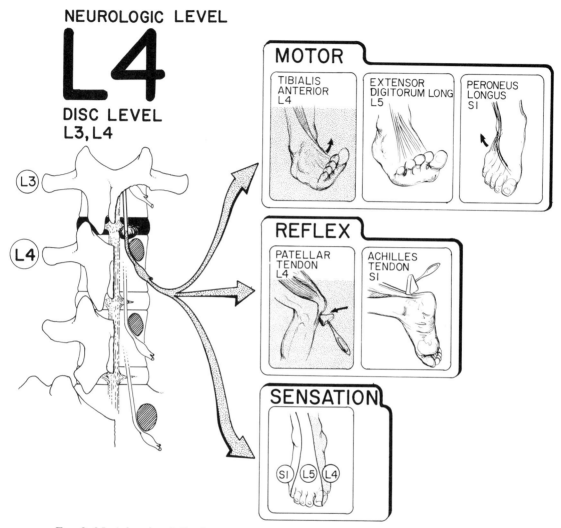

NEUROLOGIC LEVEL
L4
DISC LEVEL
L3, L4

MOTOR

TIBIALIS ANTERIOR L4 | EXTENSOR DIGITORUM LONG L5 | PERONEUS LONGUS SI

REFLEX

PATELLAR TENDON L4 | ACHILLES TENDON SI

SENSATION

SI | L5 | L4

Fig. 2–35. A herniated disc between vertebrae L3 and L4 involves the L4 nerve root.

positive findings on roentgenogram or electromyogram, conservative therapy should continue despite patient pressure for a change in treatment.

Although neurologic involvement of a herniated disc is most often manifested by the alteration of only one or two signs, there should be enough information to help pinpoint the involved neurologic level. Certainly the electromyogram and myelogram can be used as further diagnostic tools. But your clinical judgment, based on the physical examination of the patient, will most often allow you to make the proper neurologic diagnosis and prescribe the correct treatment.

Spondylolysis and Spondylolysthesis

Spondylolysis refers to the lytic line that crosses the pars interarticularis, the area between the superior and the inferior articulating processes, or, more precisely, the point at which the inferior articulating process ap-

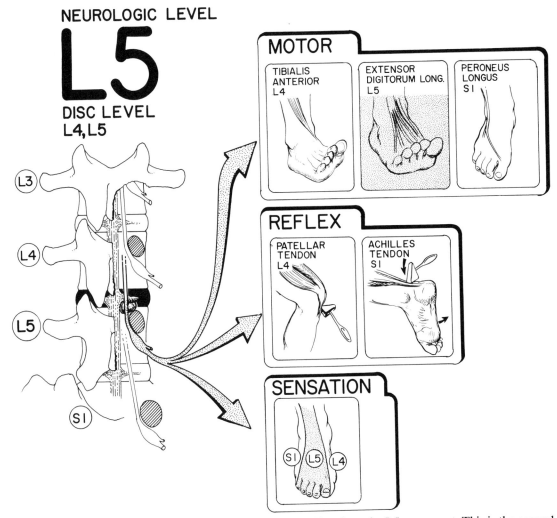

NEUROLOGIC LEVEL

L5

DISC LEVEL
L4,L5

MOTOR

TIBIALIS ANTERIOR L4

EXTENSOR DIGITORUM LONG. L5

PERONEUS LONGUS S1

REFLEX

PATELLAR TENDON L4

ACHILLES TENDON S1

SENSATION

FIG. 2–36. A herniated disc between vertebrae L4 and L5 involves the L5 nerve root. This is the second most common level of disc herniation in the lumbar spine.

proaches the pedicle. As a result of this pathology, the involved vertebra may slip forward on the vertebra immediately inferior to it. This forward slippage is called spondylolysthesis. Although the etiology of the defect of the pars interarticularis is still unknown, it is commonly believed to be the result of a fracture due to repeated stress. Because of the frequency of L5-S1 spondylolysthesis with involvement of L5-S1 nerve roots, the hamstrings, supplied medially by L5 and laterally by S1, may well go into spasm. Both sensation and reflex usually remain normal, unless there is an associated herniated disc. Occasionally, spondylolysthesis may occur even with an intact pars interarticularis in patients with degenerative arthritis. However this is very unusual.

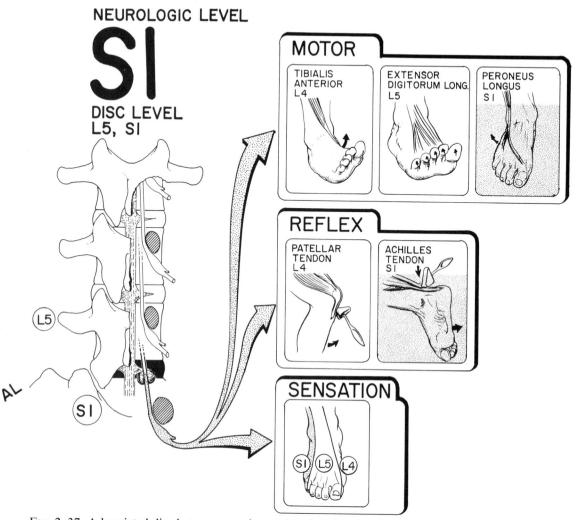

NEUROLOGIC LEVEL

S1

DISC LEVEL
L5, S1

MOTOR

TIBIALIS ANTERIOR L4

EXTENSOR DIGITORUM LONG. L5

PERONEUS LONGUS S1

REFLEX

PATELLAR TENDON L4

ACHILLES TENDON S1

SENSATION

S1 L5 L4

FIG. 2–37. A herniated disc between vertebrae L5 and S1 involves the S1 nerve root. This is the most common level of disc herniation in the lumbar spine.

The degree of forward slippage is measured clinically by the relationship of the superior vertebra to the inferior vertebra (the superior vertebra slips forward). A slip of up to 25 percent is termed a first-degree slip, 25 to 50 percent a second-degree slip, and 50 to 75 percent a third-degree slip. Any greater slippage is termed a fourth-degree slip. The vertebra most commonly involved in spondylolysis and spondylolysthesis is the L5 vertebra. The second most common is L4.

The degree of pain that the patient experiences is not necessarily related to the degree of slippage, so that a patient with a first-degree slip may feel greater pain than a patient with a fourth-degree slip, who may, in fact, feel no pain at all.

An increase of symptoms in patients with spondylolysis or spondylolysthesis can often be a result of an associated herniated lumbar disc. The incidence of a herniated disc is greater in patients with spondylolysthesis than

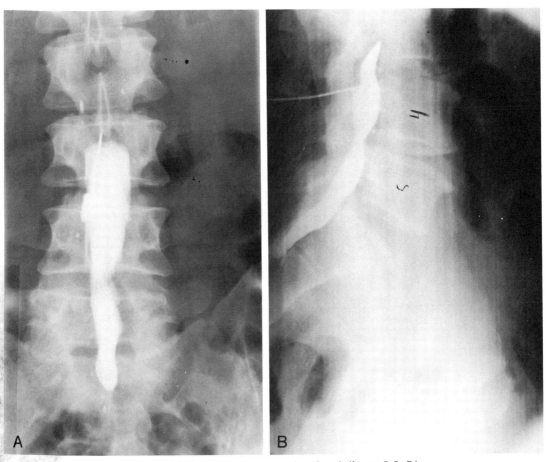

FIG. 2–38A, B. Myelogram: a herniated disc at L5, S1.

in the general population. The disc herniation usually occurs one level above the bony pathology. For example, if there is a bony defect at L5, the disc between L4 and L5 is the one most likely to herniate. The involvement of the L5 nerve root may produce associated neurologic findings, such as positive straight leg raising, toe extensor weakness, and diminution of sensation on the dorsum of the foot. Although such involvement usually stems from an associated herniation, the nerve root may also become impinged directly from a spondylolysthesis.

Spondylolysis and spondylolysthesis are frequent causes of teenage backache; the patient usually complains of back pain, particularly after sports activities.

Note that spondylolysis has a characteristic look on a roentgenogram (Fig. 2–39, 2–40).

Herpes Zoster

Herpes zoster (shingles) is a viral disease which usually involves a single, unilateral dermatome. Thoracic roots are most commonly involved. Pain frequently precedes the appearance of the skin lesion and follows the distribution of the nerve root, without crossing the midline. The level involved can be located

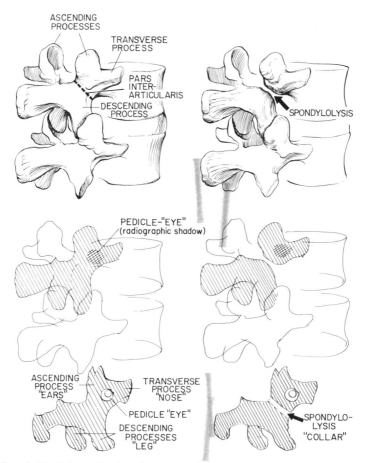

FIG. 2–39. Schematic drawing of an oblique roentgenogram of the lumbar spine, showing the characteristic "scotty dog" look of its posterior elements. Note that the defect in the pars interarticularis appears to be a collar around the dog's neck.

through appropriate sensory testing and evaluation of the level of the skin lesion.

Poliomyelitis

Poliomyelitis is an acute viral infectious disease which may inflict temporary or permanent destructive changes in motor function. It involves the destruction of the anterior horn cells of the spinal cord. Poliomyelitis usually attacks younger patients, causing motor paralysis and atrophy. It does not affect sensation, and reflexes, although diminished, are usually present, because the reflex arcs remain intact unless all the anterior horn cells are destroyed (Fig. 2–41).

Although its lesion lies in the cord, the clinical appearance of poliomyelitis may be similar to that of a nerve root lesion, since the virus destroys the cells of the nerve root. At least 50 percent of the anterior horn cells in the levels innervating a particular muscle must

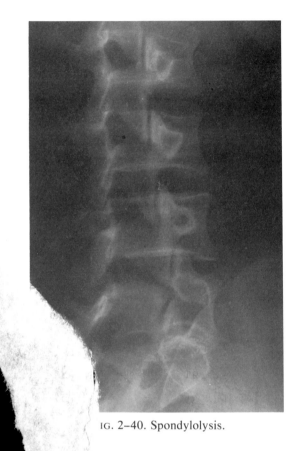

IG. 2–40. Spondylolysis.

be involved before there is any clinical evidence of muscle weakness (according to W. J. W. Sharrard). Poliomyelitis attacks the anterior horn cells segmentally – it does not simply involve all levels in an area – and it may skip levels, leaving them free of pathology. This leads to a smaller degree of involvement for muscles which are innervated by several layers. For example, the quadriceps muscle, which is innervated by L2, L3, and L4, does not experience any significant weakness unless 50 percent of the anterior horn cells of all three levels are involved. Conversely, the tibialis anterior muscle, which is innervated mainly by L4, is affected by the involvement of 50 percent of the anterior horn cells of that level, causing the relatively common problem of foot drop. If the anterior horn cells of the fifth lumbar level are involved, weakness of the gluteus medius muscle, the medial hamstrings, and the toe extensors may occur. If the anterior horn cells of the first sacral level are involved, there may be weakening of the gluteus maximus muscle, the lateral hamstring, and the peronei and calf muscles.

Through vaccination, poliomyelitis has been practically eliminated as a serious problem.

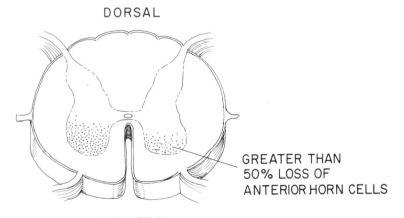

DORSAL

GREATER THAN
50% LOSS OF
ANTERIOR HORN CELLS

VENTRAL

FIG. 2–41. Anterior horn cell loss leading to clinical muscle weakness.

MUSCLE	NEUROLOGIC LEVEL*		NERVE
Hip flexors	L-1,2,3		
Hip adductors	L-2,3,4		Obturator nerve
Quadriceps	L-2,3,4		Femoral nerve
Tib. anterior	L-4,5		Deep peroneal nerve
Tib. posterior	L-4,5		Post. tibial nerve
Glut. medius	L-4,$\underline{5}$	S-1	Superior gluteal nerve
Med. hamstrings	L-4,$\underline{5}$	S-1	Sciatic nerve, tibial portion
Ex. Dig. longus	L-$\underline{5}$	S-1	Deep peroneal nerve
Ex. Hal. longus	L-$\underline{5}$	S-1	Deep peroneal nerve
Peronei	L-5	S-$\underline{1}$,2	Superficial peroneal nerve
Calf	L-5	S-$\underline{1}$,2	Tibial nerve
Lat. hamstring	L-5	S-$\underline{1}$,2	Sciatic nerve, tibial portion
Glut. maximus	L-5	S-$\underline{1}$,2	Inferior gluteal nerve
Flex. Hal. Long.	S-$\underline{1}$,2		Tibial nerve
Flex. Dig. Long.	S-1,2		Tibial nerve
Toe intrinsics	S-2,3		Lat. and Med. plantar nerves
Perineum	S-2,3,4		

*   According to Sharrard
___   Predominant neurologic level

Part Two

Spinal Cord Lesions by Neurologic Level

The acute injuries leading to tetraplegia and paraplegia present great problems in both early diagnosis of the levels of neural involvement and prognostication of future function. In today's society, where potentially debilitating occurrences, including war, auto and industrial accidents, and contact sports, are common, there is a need for a concise system of early neurologic examination. Traumatic pathology of any kind that affects the spine and spinal cord must be diagnosed immediately and must be accurately and promptly treated. The key to management of spinal injuries is immediate protection of the spinal cord, even if an immediate examination is not performed. Without immediate protection, in-complete lesions of the cord can be converted to complete lesions, and partially contused nerve roots may be totally lost.

Spinal injuries may occur at any level. Each level at which an injury can occur gives special problems: acute injuries to the cervical spine may result in death or tetraplegia; injuries to the thoracic spine usually lead to spastic paraplegia; and injuries to the lumbar spine (cauda equina injuries) can result in varying degrees of flaccid lower extremity paralysis. The following discussion deals with these three zones and with methods of examination that help to establish a precise level of neural involvement and still are economical of time and effort.

3 Cervical Cord Lesions: Tetraplegia

Tetraplegia, or quadriplegia as it is more commonly known, means paralysis involving all four extremities. The lesion which causes such paralysis occurs in the cervical spine. While it results in complete paralysis of the lower extremities, it may partially or wholly affect the upper extremities, depending upon the neurologic level involved.

In an analysis of tetraplegia, establishment of the level of neural involvement and evaluation of its degree (whether the cord lesion is complete or incomplete) are of primary concern. Both these factors must be known before there can be any attempt at prediction of recovery of neurologic function or before any effective program of therapeutic treatment and rehabilitation can be planned. The more rapid the rate of return of spinal cord function, the greater the amount of recovery and, conversely, the slower the rate of return, the smaller the amount of recovery. This rule of thumb makes it easier to estimate the future possibility of both ambulation and bladder and bowel function. Since, at the beginning, the patient may be in a state of spinal shock (diaschisis), from which some neural recovery may occur, a thorough neurologic examination, repeated every two to four hours for the first 48 hours, may begin to provide some answers about the potential for recovery. Each examination must include muscle testing, sensory testing, and

reflex testing to permit a complete evaluation of the possibility of cord return.

EVALUATION OF INDIVIDUAL CORD LEVELS: C3 TO T1

If the cervical cord is completely transected, complete paralysis of the lower extremities occurs, but the degree of paralysis of the upper extremities depends on the neurologic level involved. Although some cervical cord lesions are, in reality, incomplete or partial (so that some function remains below the level of the lesion) we shall discuss the signs as if each cord lesion is complete, since the real issue is to determine the level of injury.

Spinal shock and associated muscle flaccidity usually pass between 24 hours and three months after trauma. Spasticity and clonus set in and gradually increase in intensity. The deep tendon reflexes become exaggerated and pathologic reflexes appear.

Neurologic Level C3 (C3 Intact)

A neurologic level of C3 means that the third cervical root is intact, while the fourth is not. Neurologic level C3 corresponds to vertebral level C3-4 (Figs. 3–1, 3–2).

Motor Function. There is no motor function in the upper extremities; the patient is completely tetraplegic. Muscles are flaccid as a

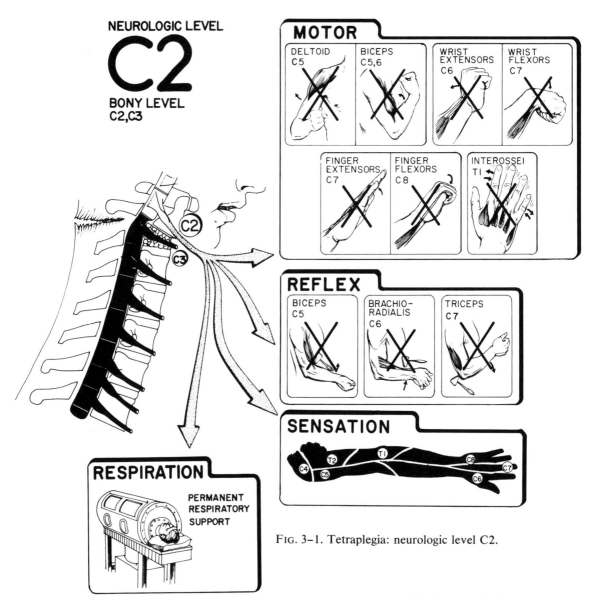

FIG. 3–1. Tetraplegia: neurologic level C2.

result of denervation and spinal shock. After spinal shock has worn off, the muscles will demonstrate varying degrees of spastic response. Since the diaphragm is supplied largely by C4, the patient is unable to breathe independently, and will die without artificial respiratory assistance. Sometimes, in what at first appears to be a C3 level, C4 later recovers, with a return of diaphragmatic function.

Sensation. There is no sensation in the upper extremities or below a line three inches above the nipple on the anterior chest wall.

Reflexes. In the presence of spinal shock, all deep tendon reflexes are absent. When spinal shock has worn off, they will become brisk to exaggerated and pathologic reflexes may be evident.

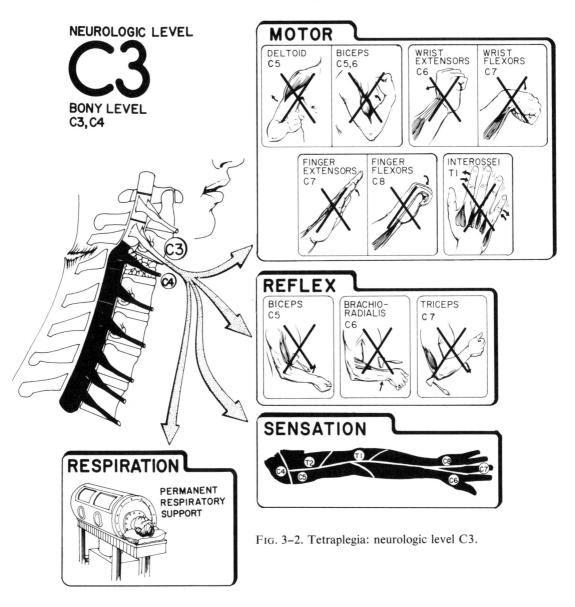

FIG. 3–2. Tetraplegia: neurologic level C3.

Neurologic Level C4 (C4 Intact)

The fourth cervical cord segment remains intact. The lesion lies between the 4th and 5th cervical vertebrae (Fig. 3–3).

Motor Function. The muscles of the upper extremity are nonfunctional. Since C4 is intact, the patient can breathe independently and shrug his shoulder. But the lack of functioning intercostal and abdominal muscles keeps the patient's respiratory reserve low, although probably adequate for the reduced level of function.

Sensation is present on the upper anterior chest wall, but not in the upper extremities.

Reflexes. Initially, all deep tendon reflexes

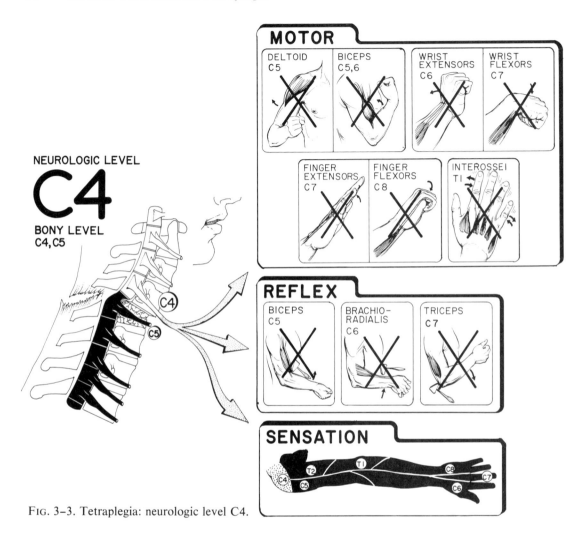

FIG. 3–3. Tetraplegia: neurologic level C4.

are absent, but the passing of spinal shock may bring changes.

Neurologic Level C5 (C5 Intact)

A lesion at this level leaves C5 intact. Since this is the first cord level to contribute to the formation of the brachial plexus, the upper extremity will have some function (Fig. 3–4).

Motor Function. The deltoid muscle and a portion of biceps muscle are functioning. The patient is able to perform shoulder abduction, flexion, and extension, as well as some elbow flexion. However, all these motions are weakened since the muscles governing these movements usually have contributions from the C6 nerve root. The patient cannot propel a wheelchair by himself and his respiratory reserve is low.

Sensation is normal over the upper portion of the anterior chest and the lateral aspect of the arm from the shoulder to the elbow crease.

Reflexes. Since the biceps reflex is primarily mediated through C5, it may be normal or slightly decreased. As spinal shock wears off

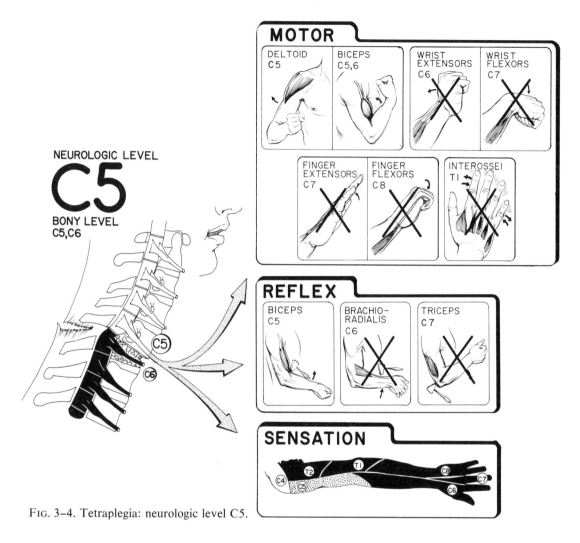

NEUROLOGIC LEVEL
C5
BONY LEVEL
C5,C6

FIG. 3–4. Tetraplegia: neurologic level C5.

and elements of C6 return, the reflex may become brisk.

Neurologic Level C6 (C6 Intact)

Involvement is at skeletal level C6-7 (Fig. 3–5).

Motor Function. Because both C5 and C6 are intact, the biceps and the rotator cuff muscles function. The most distal functional muscle group is the wrist extensor group; the extensor carpi radialis longus and brevis (C6) are both innervated (although the extensor carpi ulnaris — C7 — is still involved). The patient has almost full function of the shoulder, full flexion of the elbow, full supination and partial pronation of the forearm, and partial extension of the wrist. The strength of wrist extension is normal, since power for extension is predominantly supplied by the extensor carpi radialis longus and brevis.

Respiratory reserve is still low. The patient is confined to a wheelchair, which he can propel over smooth, level surfaces.

Sensation. The lateral side of the entire

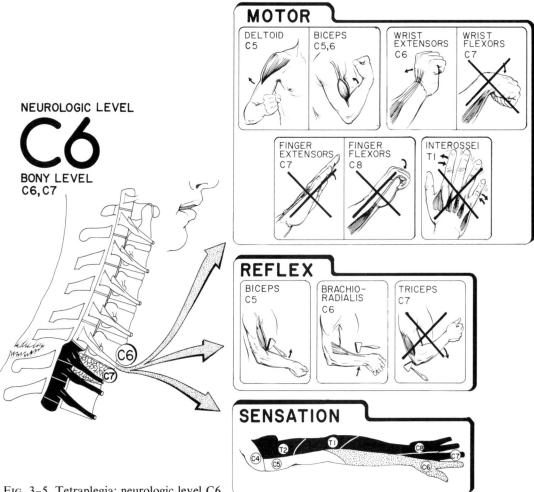

NEUROLOGIC LEVEL

C6

BONY LEVEL
C6, C7

FIG. 3–5. Tetraplegia: neurologic level C6.

upper extremity, as well as the thumb, the index, and half of the middle finger, have a normal sensory supply.

Reflexes. Both the biceps and the brachioradialis reflexes are normal.

Neurologic Level C7 (C7 Intact)

Involvement is at vertebral level C7-T1 (Fig. 3–6).

Motor Function. With the C7 nerve root intact, the triceps, the wrist flexors, and the long finger extensors are functional. The patient can hold objects, but his grasp is extremely weak. Although he is still confined to a wheelchair, the patient may begin to attempt parallel bar and brace ambulation for general exercise.

Sensation. C7 has little pure sensory representation in the upper extremity. No precise zone for C7 sensation has been mapped.

Reflexes. The biceps (C5), brachioradialis (C6), and triceps (C7) reflexes are normal.

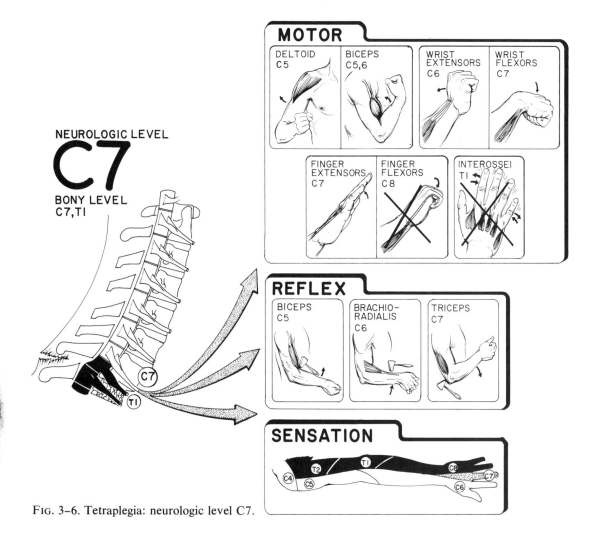

FIG. 3–6. Tetraplegia: neurologic level C7.

Neurologic Level C8 (C8 Intact)

Involvement is at skeletal level T1-T2 (Fig. 3–7).

Motor Function. The upper extremity is normal, except for the intrinsics of the hand. Thus, all upper extremity motions except finger abduction, finger adduction, and the pinch mechanism of the thumb, index, and middle fingers are intact. Grasp is difficult, since the hand is intrinsic minus or clawed.

Sensation. The lateral aspect of the upper extremity and the entire hand have normal sensory awareness. Sensation on the medial side of the forearm is normal to several inches below the elbow.

Reflexes. All upper extremity reflexes are intact.

Neurologic Level T1 (T1 Intact)

Involvement occurs at skeletal level T2-T3.

Motor Function. Involvement at neurologic level T1 results in paraplegia. The upper extremity is fully functional. The brachial plexus' neurologic supply (C5-T1) is intact, while the lower extremities are partially or

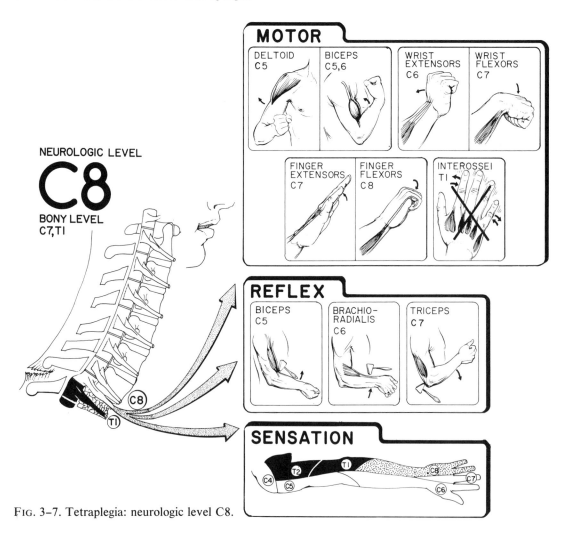

NEUROLOGIC LEVEL

C8

BONY LEVEL
C7, T1

FIG. 3–7. Tetraplegia: neurologic level C8.

wholly paralyzed, depending upon the degree of cord damage at that level. The patient can ambulate in a variety of ways with correct bracing, but a wheelchair is still the most practical means of moving about. A T1 paraplegic can drag-to with crutches and bracing but he cannot assume the erect position without some help. Trunk stability is absent, and the energy cost of ambulation is markedly increased. Therefore, ambulation is not functional, but is useful as exercise.

Sensation. The anterior chest wall as low as the nipple and the entire upper extremity have normal sensation.

Reflexes. The reflexes in the upper extremity are normal.

Upper Motor Neuron Reflexes

Pathologic reflexes appear in the upper and lower extremities in association with tetraplegia. Hoffmann's sign can be elicited in the upper extremity and, if present, is an indication of an upper motor neuron lesion.

To test for Hoffmann's sign, nip the nail of

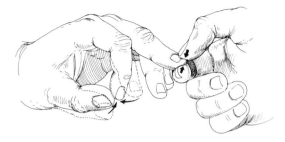

FIG. 3-8. Hoffmann's sign, indicating an upper motor neuron lesion.

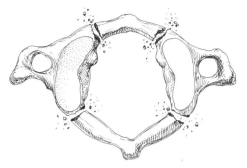

FIG. 3-9. Jefferson fracture, a bursting fracture of the ring of C1.

the middle finger. Normally there should be no reaction at all. A positive reaction produces flexion of the terminal phalanx of the thumb and of the second and third phalanx of another finger (Fig. 3-8).

CLINICAL APPLICATION

Fractures and Dislocations of the Cervical Spine

Injuries to the cervical spine are a major cause of tetraplegia. The types of injury include flexion injuries (compression fractures), hyperextension injuries, and flexion-rotation injuries (cervical facet dislocations).

On occasion, the neurologic level involved does not correspond to the skeletal level. Thus, in a fracture-dislocation of the 5th and 6th cervical vertebrae, the C6 neurologic level may remain functional. Each patient must be evaluated on an individual basis.

Fracture of C1. The C1 or Jefferson fracture is a bursting fracture of the ring of C1, which usually decompresses the cord. The fracture commonly results from a fall, with the patient landing on his head. If the patient survives, there are usually no permanent neurologic findings (Fig. 3-9, 3-10).

Fracture of C2. The C2 or hangman's fracture is a bursting fracture that separates the body of C2 from its posterior elements, thereby decompressing the cord. If the patient sur-

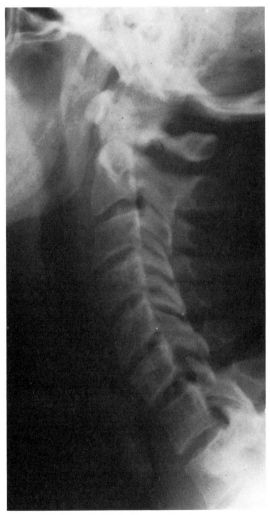

FIG. 3-10. Jefferson fracture.

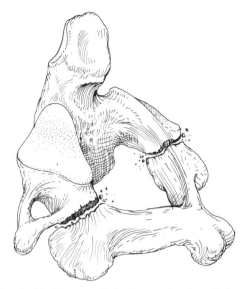

FIG. 3–11. Hangman's fracture, a fracture that separates the body of C2 from its posterior elements.

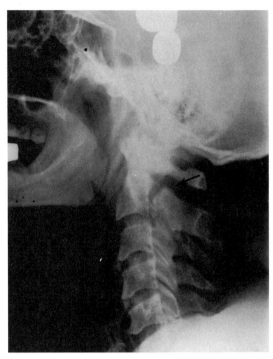

FIG. 3–12. Hangman's fracture.

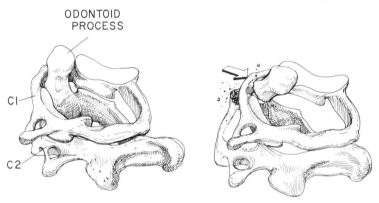

FIG. 3–13. Odontoid fracture.

vives, there are usually only transient neurologic findings (Fig. 3–11, 3–12).

Odontoid Fracture. A fracture at the base of the odontoid commonly results from trauma. The patient usually survives. There may be transient neurologic findings, but without the establishment of the involvement of a specific neurologic level. On occasion, if the trauma is severe enough, the patient dies. However, there is usually enough space in the cervical canal to allow for partial displacement of the odontoid (Fig. 3–13, 3–14).

Fractures of C3-C7

COMPRESSION FRACTURES are caused by hyperflexion injuries of the neck when a vertical force ruptures the end plates of the ver-

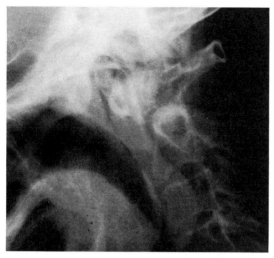

FIG. 3–14. Odontoid fracture.

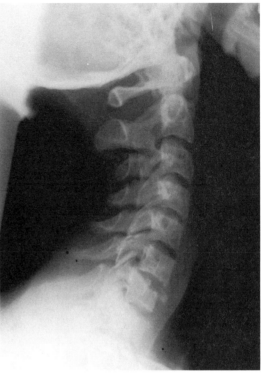

FIG. 3–16. Cervical spine compression fracture.

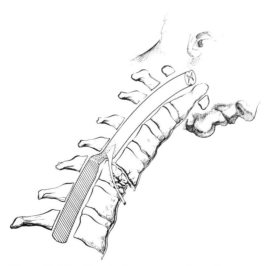

FIG. 3–15. Cervical compression fracture, caused by hyperflexion of the neck.

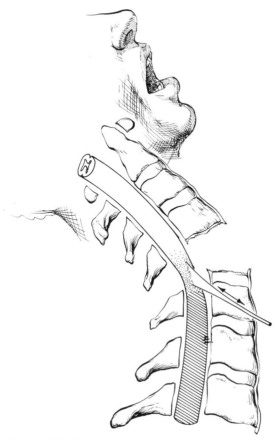

FIG. 3–17. Hyperextension injury of the cervical spine.

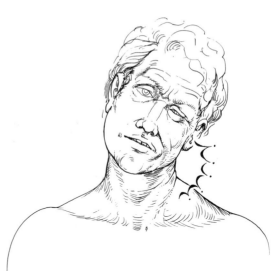

FIG. 3–18. Pain associated with facet joint dislocation.

tebra and shatters the body. This bursting fracture occurs in both the cervical and lumbar spines and may involve both the nerve root and the cord itself (Fig. 3–15). A compression fracture of the C5 vertebra, the most common fracture of the cervical spine, involves most of the brachial plexus and may result in tetraplegia. Compression fractures are easy to diagnose on roentgenograms (Fig. 3–16).

HYPEREXTENSION INJURIES of the neck are caused by hyperextension forces, such as the acceleration injury caused by a rear-end automobile collision. A hyperextension injury is essentially a soft tissue injury, unlike a compression injury, which fractures the body of the vertebra; the anterior longitudinal ligament is usually ruptured and the cord may well become involved. Because it is a soft tissue injury, the hyperextension injury may not be obvious on roentgenograms (Fig. 3–17).

CERVICAL FACET JOINT DISLOCATIONS are flexion-rotation injuries which may cause neurologic problems. A unilateral facet dislocation produces some narrowing of the spinal canal and neural foramen. Because a unilateral facet dislocation usually results in less than 50 percent anterior dislocation of the vertebral body, approximately 75 percent of cases have no neurologic involvement, since the narrowing is not sufficient to affect the cord. (Figs. 3–18, 3–21).

BILATERAL FACET DISLOCATIONS produce far greater narrowing of the spinal canal than unilateral dislocations since, with both facets dislocated, there is usually greater than 50 percent anterior dislocation of the vertebral body. Because of this greater degree of dislocation, approximately 85 percent of patients suffer neurologic lesions. Because the cervical spine depends primarily on ligaments for its stability, bilateral facet dislocations, which

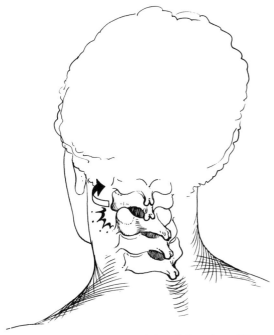

FIG. 3–19. Unilateral facet joint dislocation. (Hoppenfeld, S.: Physical Examination of the Spine and Extremities, Appleton-Century-Crofts.)

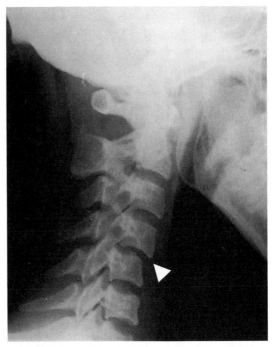

FIG. 3–21. Unilateral facet joint dislocation.

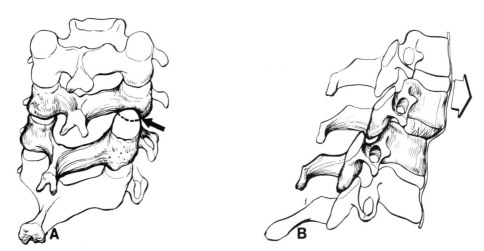

FIG. 3–20A, B. In a unilateral facet joint dislocation, there is less than 50 per cent anterior dislocation of the vertebral body.

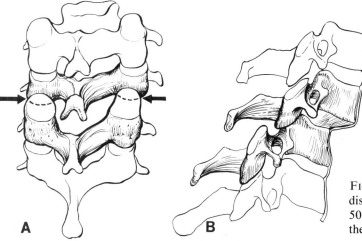

A   **B**

Fig. 3–22A, B. Bilateral facet joint dislocation, resulting in greater than 50 per cent anterior dislocation of the vertebral body.

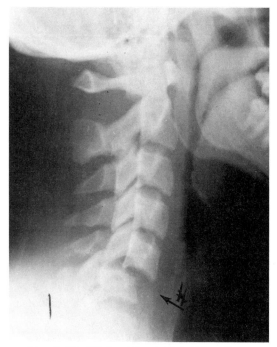

Fig. 3–23. Bilateral facet joint dislocation.

cause the ligaments to tear, rarely heal with sufficient strength to reinstate spinal stability; unless appropriate treatment is undertaken, there is a risk of further damage secondary to any number of possible accidents. Bilateral

dislocations may occur at any level, but they are most common at C5-C6, the level around which the most movement takes place (except for the specialized articulation at C1-C2) (Fig. 3–22, 3–23).

Activities of Daily Living

Respiration. From the above description of cord lesions, it should be apparent that a complete transection of the cord at neurologic level C3 or higher is incompatible with life, unless the patient is permanently ventilated. Involvement at neurologic levels C4 to C5 may cause degrees of respiratory insufficiency that may threaten life in the presence of relatively mild pulmonary disease.

Wheelchair. C6 is the highest neurologic level that leaves sufficient innervation of the upper extremity to permit independent manipulation of a wheelchair. However, independent transfer into and out of the wheelchair is still difficult because of the lack of function of the triceps muscle. An active triceps is needed to help lift the body for transfer.

Crutches. Complete cord lesions at neurologic level C8 and above are incompatible with the use of crutches since the intrinsic muscles of the hand, needed for strong grip on the crutches, are nonfunctioning. Functional

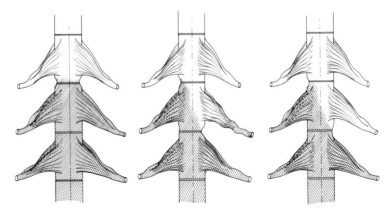

Fig. 3–24. The findings resulting from a complete lesion depend upon the anatomic configuration of the destruction of neural tissue at a particular level.

walking with crutches is made more difficult both because of the need to expend two to four times more energy than in normal ambulation and because of a decreased respiratory reserve. Attempts to encourage walking with braces and other supports are also rarely successful.

Note that the above is true of complete cord lesions; partial cord lesions show varying patterns of neurologic deficiency. Each patient must be assessed as an individual (Fig. 3–24).

Herniated Cervical Discs

Although herniated cervical discs often cause neurologic root involvement, the cervical canal is sufficiently large to accommodate the herniated disc without significant cord damage, and tetraplegia rarely occurs. However, minor degrees of cord damage—upper motor neuron lesions—may result from a large midline herniation. They are usually first recognized as a diminution in sensation of position and vibration in the lower extremities. In more advanced cases, there may be actual muscle weakness and an increase in the deep tendon reflexes, as well as early bladder symptoms.

Tumors of the Cervical Spine

Tumors of the cervical cord are space-occupying lesions. They may present as local pain in the spine, and may also radiate pain into the extremities. The anatomic location of the tumor can usually be ascertained by a neurologic evaluation of the extremity. For example, a tumor of the cervical cord involving the C6-C7 neurologic segment may cause anesthesia of the middle finger, an absence of the triceps reflex, and weakness of finger extension and wrist flexion. Primary tumors of the cord rarely give precise neurologic levels of involvement.

Metastatic tumors in the vertebrae of the cervical spine are not uncommon. Primary breast and lung tumors frequently metastasize to the spine. As bone is destroyed, vertebral collapse and angulation take place and tetraplegia occurs. The neurologic level of involvement usually correlates with the x-ray findings.

Tuberculosis of the Spine

Tuberculosis of the spine causes gibbus formation through the destruction of bone. The spinal angulation may ultimately cause cord compression and tetraplegia, but the process is far slower than that of trauma. Frequently, neurologic recovery occurs after surgical decompression and chemotherapy.

Transverse Myelitis

Transverse myelitis refers to an inflammatory process in which a spinal cord lesion extending horizontally across the cord is limited longitudinally to one or, at most, a few spinal segments. Ascending myelitis occurs when the lesion spreads proximally.

Transverse myelitis may occur spontaneously and rapidly following a vaccination, an infectious illness, or trauma. Although sensory and motor loss occurs below the lesion, complete anesthesia is rare. Flaccid paralysis occurs initially, but quickly reverts to spastic paralysis.

The neurologic level of involvement can usually be delineated by neurologic level testing of sensation, motor power, and reflexes. The highest level of sensory loss usually corresponds to the segmental site of the cord lesion.

4 Spinal Cord Lesions Below T1, Including the Cauda Equina

PARAPLEGIA

Paraplegia is the complete or partial paralysis of the lower extremities and lower portion of the body. It is most frequently caused by traumatic injury to the spine, but may also derive from various diseases, such as transverse myelitis, cystic lesions of the cord, and Pott's paraplegia (caused by tuberculosis), as well as a host of other pathologies. It occurs rarely from surgical correction of such thoracic problems as scoliosis, as a result of the loss of the appropriate blood supply to the spinal cord, and from the excision of a herniated thoracic disc.

Below L1, the cauda equina begins; lesions in this area, called cauda equina injuries, rarely result in full paralysis of the lower extremities.

The following descriptions assume that a complete lesion exists. Often, however, lesions are incomplete; the neurologic findings for each individual patient must be carefully determined, for involvement may vary considerably.

Neurologic Levels T1 to T12

The level of neurologic involvement can be determined by tests of motor power and sensation. The latter is easier and more accurate.

Muscle Function. The intercostal muscles, as well as the abdominal and paraspinal muscles, are segmentally innervated. Intercostal motion during breathing implies neurologic integrity; a lack of motion implies involvement. The abdominal and paraspinal muscles can be similarly evaluated, for they are both segmentally innervated by T7 to T12 (L1). To test for the integrity of their innervation, have the patient do a half sit up as you palpate the anterior abdominal wall. As the patient sits up, note whether the umbilicus is pulled toward any of the four quadrants of the abdomen. If the umbilicus is pulled in one direction, the opposing flaccid muscles are denervated (Beevor sign) (Fig. 2–1). Note that the umbilicus is the dividing line between T10 above and T11 below. Obviously, this test should not be performed during the acute stages of thoracic lesions or with patients who have unstable spines.

Sensation. Sensory innervation may be determined in accordance with the chart (Fig. 4–1). Special skin landmarks that mark sensory areas are:

1. Nipple line – T4
2. Xiphoid process – T7
3. Umbilicus – T10
4. Groin – T12

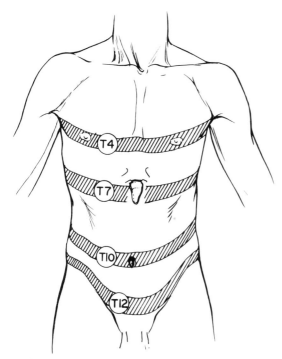

FIG. 4–1. Sensory dermatomes of the trunk.

L1 Neurologic Level (L1 Intact)

Muscle Function. There is complete paralysis of the lower extremities, with the exception of some hip flexion from partial innervation of the iliopsoas (T12, L1, 2, 3).

Sensation. There is no sensation below the L1 sensory band, which extends over the proximal third of the anterior aspect of the thigh.

Reflexes. The patellar and Achilles tendon reflexes are absent when spinal shock is present. As spinal shock wears off, the reflexes become exaggerated.

Bladder and Bowel Function. The bladder (S2, 3, 4) does not function. The patient cannot urinate in a stream. The anus is initially patulous, and the superficial anal reflex (S2, 3, 4) is absent. As spinal shock wears off, the anal sphincter contracts and the anal reflex becomes hyperactive.

L2 Neurologic Level (L2 Intact)

Muscle Function. There is good power in hip flexion because the iliopsoas is almost completely innervated. The adductor muscles are partially innervated (L2, 3, 4) and show diminished power. Although the quadriceps (L2, 3, 4) are partially innervated, there is no clinically significant function. No other muscles in the lower extremity have innervation, and the unopposed action of the iliopsoas and adductors tends to produce a flexion and slight adduction deformity.

Sensation. There is no sensation below the L2 sensory band, which ends two-thirds of the way down the thigh.

Reflexes. The patellar reflex receives innervation from L2, 3, and 4, but the L2 contribution is small.

Bladder and Bowel Function. There is no voluntary control.

L3 Neurologic Level (L3 Intact)

Muscle Function. In addition to the iliopsoas and adductors, the quadriceps, although slightly weak, (L2, 3, 4) show significant power. No other muscle groups are functioning. Thus, the hip tends to become flexed, adducted, and externally rotated, while the knee remains extended.

Sensation. Sensation is normal to the level of the knee (L3 dermatome band).

Reflexes. The patellar reflex (L2, 3, *4*) is present, but decreased. The Achilles tendon reflex is absent.

Bladder and Bowel Function. There is no voluntary control.

L4 Neurologic Level (L4 Intact)

Muscle Function. Muscle function at the hip and knee is the same as in L3 neurologic lesions except that quadriceps function is now normal. The only functioning muscle below the knee is the tibialis anterior (L4), which causes the foot to dorsiflex and invert.

Sensation. In addition to the entire thigh, the medial side of the tibia and foot have sensation.

Reflexes. The patellar reflex (predominantly L4) is normal; the Achilles tendon reflex (S1) is still absent.

Bladder and Bowel Function. There is no voluntary control of either function.

L5 Neurologic Level (L5 Intact)

Muscle Function. The hip still has a flexion deformity, because the gluteus maximus does not function. The gluteus medius (L1-S1) has partial function; it counteracts the action of the adductors. The quadriceps are normal.

The knee flexors function partially with the medial hamstrings (L5) present and the lateral hamstrings (S1) absent.

The foot dorsiflexors and invertors function. Since the plantar-flexors and evertors are still absent, the foot tends to develop a calcaneus (dorsiflexion) deformity.

Sensation. Sensation is normal in the lower extremity, with the exception of the lateral side and plantar surface of the foot.

Reflexes. The patellar reflex is normal. The Achilles tendon reflex is still absent.

Bladder and Bowel Function. There is no voluntary control of either function.

S1 Neurologic Level (S1 Intact)

Muscle Function. The hip muscles are normal, with the exception of slight gluteus maximus weakness. The knee muscles are normal. The soleus and gastrocnemius (S1, 2) are weak, and the toes show clawing as a result of intrinsic muscle weakness (S2, 3).

Sensation. Sensation in the lower extremity is normal. There is perianal anesthesia.

Reflexes. The patellar and Achilles tendon reflexes are normal, since the S2 contribution to the Achilles tendon reflex is small.

Bladder and Bowel Function. There is still no voluntary control of either function.

UPPER MOTOR NEURON REFLEXES

Pathologic Reflexes

Pathologic reflexes can be elicited in the lower extremities in association with paraplegia. Babinski's sign and Oppenheim's sign are two pathologic reflexes which indicate an upper motor neuron lesion.

Babinski's Sign. Elicit the plantar response by running a sharp instrument across the plantar surface of the foot, and along the calcaneus and lateral border of the forefoot. Normally, in a negative reaction, the toes plantarflex. A positive reaction (Babinski's sign) occurs when the great toe extends as the other toes splay (Fig. 4-2). This sign indicates an upper motor neuron lesion—a corticospinal tract involvement. To ascertain the level of the lesion, correlate this sign with other neurologic findings. In young infants, the presence of Babinski's sign is normal rather than pathologic. However, this response should disappear by 12 to 18 months of age.

Oppenheim's Sign. To elicit Oppenheim's sign, run your finger along the crest of the tibia. Normally there should be no reaction at all, or the patient should complain of pain. Under abnormal circumstances, the reaction is the same as it is in plantar stimulation: the great toe extends as the other toes splay (Oppenheim's sign) (Fig. 4-3). Oppenheim's sign is not as reliable as Babinski's sign and should be used as a confirmation of a positive Babinski's sign.

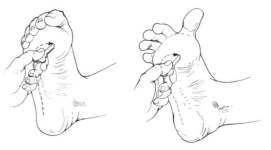

Fig. 4-2. Babinski's sign.

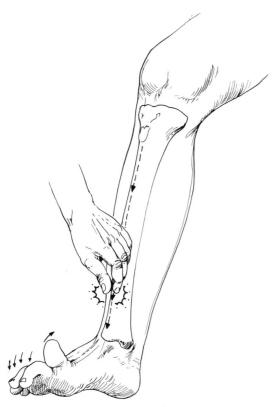

FIG. 4–3. Oppenheim's sign.

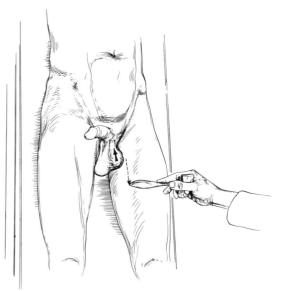

FIG. 4–4. The cremasteric reflex. (Hoppenfeld, S.: Physical Examination of the Spine and Extremities, Appleton-Century-Crofts.)

Normal Superficial Reflex

Cremasteric. The lack of the cremasteric reflex may be due either to the loss of the reflex arc or to an upper motor neuron lesion. However, absence of the reflex in association with the presence of a pathologic reflex (Babinski's or Oppenheim's signs) supports the diagnosis of an upper motor neuron lesion.

To elicit the superficial cremasteric reflex, stroke the inner side of the upper thigh with the sharp end of a neurologic hammer. If the reflex is intact, the scrotal sac on that side will be pulled upwards as the cremaster muscle (T12) contracts. If the cremasteric reflex is unilaterally absent, there is probably a lower motor neuron lesion between L1 and L2 (Fig. 4–4).

CLINICAL APPLICATION

Further Evaluation of Spinal Cord Injuries

Complete or Incomplete Lesion. The possibility of cord return, and whatever partial functional recovery it may provide, depends upon whether the lesion is complete or incomplete, whether the cord is completely severed or only partially severed or contused. Injuries in which no function returns over a 24-hour period are assumed to be complete lesions where no return of cord function will occur. A complete neurologic examination is needed to confirm such a diagnosis. If, however, there is partial return of function in the initial period, the lesion is probably incomplete, and more function may eventually return. Function must return at more than one neurologic level to support such a diagnosis, however, since return at only one level may simply indicate that the nerve root at the level of the lesion has

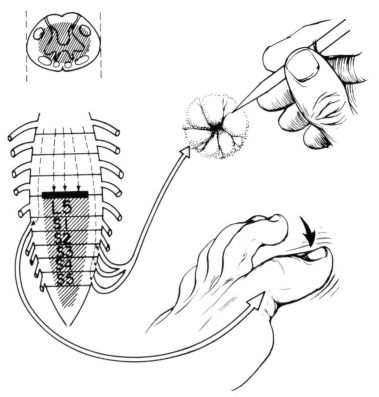

FIG. 4–5. Sacral sparing.

been partially damaged or contused. Such single level return gives no indication as to whether the lesion below it is complete or incomplete. The recovery of this single nerve root is considered to be a root lesion (rather than a cord lesion) of the root originating just proximal to the injured portion of the cord. Functional return of muscle strength from such an injury may occur at any time; prognostication for root return is good as late as six months after the initial injury.

Sacral Sparing. The best indicator of the possibility of cord return is sacral sparing, in which the sacral nerves are partially or wholly spared injury because of their location on the periphery of the cord. Evidence of sacral sparing is evidence of an incomplete lesion. It enhances the possibility of partial or complete

return of motor power as well as of bladder and bowel function.

Sacral sparing can be evaluated through three tests of motor, sensory, and reflex innervation:

1. Muscle testing of flexion of the great toe (S1 innervation)
2. Sensory testing of the perianal area (S2, 3, 4)
3. Reflex testing of the anal sphincter muscle (S2, 3, 4)

Since the bladder and bowel are innervated by the sacral nerves (S2, 3, 4), testing of these three areas gives a valid indication of the degree of sacral sparing and the possibility of return of function (Fig. 4–5).

Flaccidity and Spasticity. Immediately after any trauma causing tetraplegia or paraplegia, the spinal cord experiences spinal shock, resulting in the loss of reflexes innervated by the portion of the cord below the site of the lesion. The direct result of spinal shock is that all the muscles innervated by the traumatized portion of the cord and the portion below the lesion, as well as the bladder, become *flaccid*. Spinal shock wears off between 24 hours and three months after injury, and *spasticity* may replace flaccidity in some or all of these muscles. Spasticity occurs because the reflex arc to the muscle remains anatomically intact despite the loss of cerebral innervation and control via the long tracts. During spinal shock, the arc does not function; as the spine recovers from shock, the reflex arc begins functioning without the inhibitory or regulatory impulses from the brain, creating local spasticity and clonus. Initially absent deep tendon reflexes may therefore become hyperactive as spinal shock ends. Such spasticity may be useful in increasing function by, for example, assisting in emptying the bladder and bowel.

Prognostication of Ambulatory Function. Thoracic lesions, if they are complete, create similar problems regardless of the level of involvement. Since the thoracic cord does not supply innervation to any extremity, a complete thoracic lesion at any level leaves the patient paraplegic. The major diagnostic consideration in determining the neurologic level is that of sensory innervation to the trunk and, to a lesser extent, innervation of the abdominal musculature. In prognosticating the patient's future performance, it is important to assess the function of the segmentally innervated abdominal and paraspinal muscles that aid in balance for sitting, standing, and walking during rehabilitation.

T1 TO T8. In general, whereas a paraplegic with a lesion anywhere from T1 to T8 can be independent in all wheelchair activities, the more complex motions, such as getting up from the floor and curb jumping with a wheelchair, are more difficult for those with lesions from T1 to T4.

T6. A T6 paraplegic has complete upper extremity and thoracic musculature, and can stabilize himself against his pectoral girdle.

T9 TO T12. A paraplegic with a lesion from T9 to T12 can walk independently with long leg braces and crutches.

L1 TO L3. A paraplegic with a lesion from L1 to L3 and pelvic stability can ambulate with long leg braces and forearm crutches if he wishes.

L4 TO S2. A paraplegic with a lesion from L4 to S2 can exist independent of his wheelchair using short leg braces and forearm crutches. He is completely independent in all activities.

Although paraplegia may result from a lesion located anywhere from T1 to L1, the most common site for a lesion is between T12 and L1. The facet joints between T12 and L1 are lumbar in nature and face laterally, while those between the other thoracic vertebrae are thoracic in nature, and face vertically (Fig. 4–6). Thus, the angle between the facet joints of T12 and L1 is in the sagittal plane, permitting more flexion than the frontal alignment of the thoracic joints. Many of the other thoracic vertebrae are further limited in their motion by the rib cage. This greater concentration of motion at the T12-L1 articulations leads to a point of stress and a greater potential for fracture and subsequent paraplegia (see Fig. 4–13).

Note that there is very little room in the spinal canal at this level; any vertebral dislocation is almost certain to cause neurologic problems as a result of direct pressure on the cord. Extreme flexion and rotation is the cause of fracture-dislocation of the thoracic spine, and usually leads to paraplegia.

Prognostication of Bladder and Bowel Function. Restoring useful function to the bladder and bowel and thus a catheter-free state is crucial for tetraplegic and paraplegic patients. A bladder which must be regularly emptied through a catheter is prey to repeated infections and excessive autonomic dysreflexia

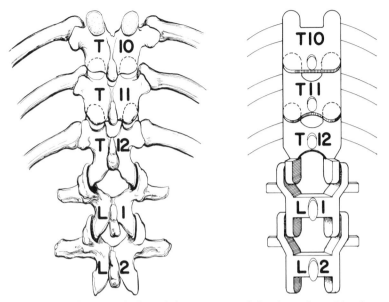

Fig. 4–6. Differences in facet joint anatomy of the thoracic and lumbar spines.

(resulting from distention of the bladder, among other peripheral stimuli) causing paroxysmal hypertension, bradycardia, and nonthermoregulatory sweating. Evaluating the extent of sacral sparing may give a clue to the possible return of function. Usually, when innervation of the bladder and its central mechanisms is intact, voiding function rapidly returns to normal. If function is only partially disrupted, a residual neurogenic disorder can be restored to useful function fairly quickly by retraining.

INCOMPLETE LESIONS. An incomplete lesion may affect the bladder and bowel in various ways. If voluntary flexion of the great toe is present, perianal sensation is intact, and there is voluntary contraction of the anal sphincter muscle, the entire sacral innervation to the bladder and bowel has probably been spared and voluntary bladder and bowel function will return, usually within a few days (Fig. 4–5).

If perianal sensation is normal and there is no voluntary contraction of the anal sphincter,

the sacral segments may have suffered partial damage (partial sacral sparing); bladder and bowel function may undergo only partial recovery.

COMPLETE LESION. A complete lesion with no sacral sparing has great influence on bladder and bowel functions. First, voluntary flexion of the great toe, perianal sensation, and voluntary sphincter control are absent, indicating permanent loss of central control of bladder and bowel function. Second, the perianal sphincter reflex (anal wink) and the bulbocavernosus reflex (in which a squeeze of the glans penis stimulates an anal sphincter contraction) (Fig. 4–7) may be present to indicate that reflex innervation of the bladder and bowel is intact. The bladder can be expected to contract on a reflex basis, and the bowel will empty as a result of a reflex induced by fecal bulb or by a rectal glycerine suppository.

It is rare that all reflexes remain absent after the initial period of spinal shock, resulting in an atonic bladder, constipation, and ileus.

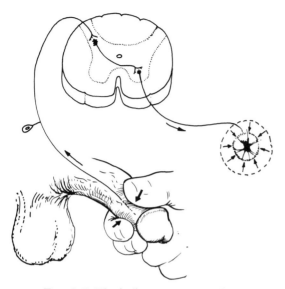

FIG. 4–7. The bulbocavernosus reflex

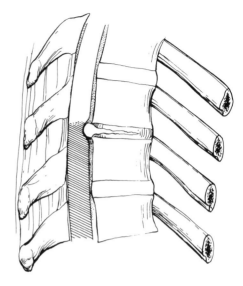

FIG. 4–8. A herniated thoracic disc.

During the atonic period, the bladder cannot contract by reflex action and must be catheterized or emptied by manual pressure on the lower abdomen. To empty the bowel will require enemas as well as manual evacuation if the stool is inspissated. As the atonic phase passes, the bladder begins to contract reflexly, and the patient can be trained to empty it by using its reflex action.

Herniated Thoracic Discs

The thoracic spine has the advantage of attachment to the ribs and sternal plate, which splint the vertebrae and provide added stability. With less motion, there is less chance for disc herniation and fracture and subsequent neurologic problems. Thus, thoracic herniated discs are rare in comparison to cervical and lumbar herniated discs.

Herniated thoracic discs usually produce *cord* involvement, while lumbar and cervical discs usually produce *nerve root* involvement. Because there is little extradural space in the thoracic spinal canal, a comparatively small disc protrusion may have pronounced effects

on the neurology (Fig. 4–8). It is more difficult to make a clinical diagnosis of a herniated thoracic disc than a herniated cervical or lumbar disc. Although evaluation of muscle power, reflexes, sensation, and bladder and bowel function can assist in determining the level of involvement, the myelogram is the cornerstone for establishing the diagnosis. Note that with herniated thoracic discs paraplegia occasionally occurs.

Motor power is impaired, but not in a myotomal or neurologic pattern. Proximal and distal muscle groups are equally weak, and leg weakness may be unilateral or bilateral. Weakness of the lower abdominal muscles may be apparent, a situation which can be evaluated by Beevor's sign (see page 45). Muscle weakness may vary from mild paresis to complete paraplegia. Muscle tone is increased in most patients, as one would expect in an upper motor neuron lesion.

Sensation. Examination can determine the level of sensory involvement. Usually it is one or two levels lower than the bony level depicted on a myelogram.

Reflexes. Deep tendon reflexes: patellar and

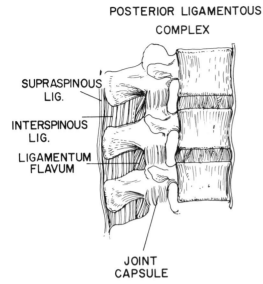

FIG. 4–9. The posterior ligamentous complex.

Achilles tendon reflexes are increased, brisk, or exaggerated.

Superficial reflexes: abdominal and cremasteric reflexes are absent.

Pathologic reflexes: Babinski's and Oppenheim's signs are usually present (Fig. 4–2, 4–3).

Bladder and Bowel Function. Most patients have no bladder or bowel symptoms. Occasionally, a patient may experience urinary retention.

It should be clear from the above discussion that the signs vary depending upon the extent of the herniation. The variations themselves may be a tip-off to the diagnosis.

EVALUATION OF SPINAL STABILITY TO PREVENT FURTHER NEUROLOGIC LEVEL INVOLVEMENT

After spinal trauma, it is crucial to determine whether the spine is stable or unstable in order to protect the spinal cord. If the spine is unstable, it must be stabilized immediately to prevent further damage to the cord, and possi-

ble tetraplegia and paraplegia. The name of the game is to protect the spinal cord.

Diagnosis

The diagnosis of an unstable spine is based on the history of the mechanism of injury, the physical examination, and an x-ray examination. Stability depends essentially on the integrity of the posterior ligamentous complex, which consists of:

1. Supraspinous ligament
2. Interspinous ligament
3. Facet joint capsule
4. Ligamentum flavum (Fig. 4–9).

The breakdown of this ligamentous complex can be diagnosed by specific criteria as shown in Table 4–1.

Roentgenography, the cornerstone of the diagnosis of instability, shows whether there is separation of the spinous processes, dislocation of the articular processes, and fracture.

Physical examination determines whether there is a palpable spinal defect (Fig. 4–10).

History may establish whether the injury was caused by flexion-rotation or excessive flexion. Direct longitudinal pull rarely ruptures fibers of the posterior ligamentous com-

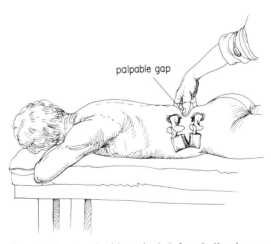

FIG. 4–10. A palpable spinal defect indicating an unstable spinal injury.

TABLE 4–1. CRITERIA FOR STABILITY OF SPINE

History of Mechanism of Injury	Physical and Neurologic Examinations	X-ray Examination Specific Criteria
Flexion-rotation Excessive flexion	Palpable spine defect Motor/reflex/sensation alteration Abrasions on the back	Spinous process separation Articular process dislocation and/or fracture
Disruption of posterior ligamentous complex	Disruption of posterior ligamentous complex	Disruption of posterior ligamentous complex

TABLE 4–2. CRITERIA FOR STABILITY OF CERVICAL SPINE

History of Mechanism of Injury	Stability	Integrity of Posterior Long. Ligament Complex	Physical Examination Neurologic Findings (N.F.)	Palpable Spine Defect (P.S.D.)	X-ray Findings
Flexion	Stable	Intact	Occasional N.F.	P.S.D.	Vertebral body crush or dislocation
Excessive flexion	Unstable	Not intact	Occasional N.F.		
Extension	Stable	Intact	Occasional N.F.	None	None
Flexion-rotation	Unilateral: stable Bilateral: unstable	Not intact	N.F.	P.S.D.	Facet dislocation

plex. However, direct longitudinal pull combined with rotation frequently ruptures fibers and results in spinal instability. Ligamentous healing is simply not strong enough to ensure spinal stability: a spine fusion is almost always necessary. If the fracture-dislocation does not disrupt the posterior ligamentous complex, bone healing is usually strong enough to ensure stability.

Flexion Injury

If, during flexion injury, the posterior ligament and complex remains intact, the force of flexion is spent on vertebral body, and a wedge compression fracture occurs. The ver-

tebral end plates remain intact, and the spinous processes are only minimally separated. A wedge compression fracture is most often seen in the cervical and lumbar spines, and is considered a stable fracture; the bone fragments are firmly impacted and the posterior ligamentous complex, including the anterior and posterior longitudinal ligaments, remains intact (Fig. 4–11).

Excessive flexion results in tearing of the posterior ligamentous complex and disengagement of the posterior facet joints, leading to pure dislocation. The spinous processes are separated, and the vertebral bodies remain uncrushed since there is no fulcrum around

FLEXION INJURY
STABLE

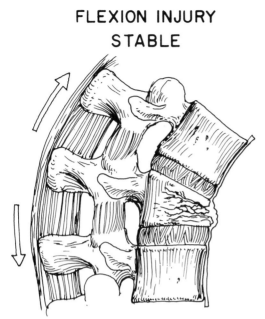

FIG. 4–11. A flexion injury.

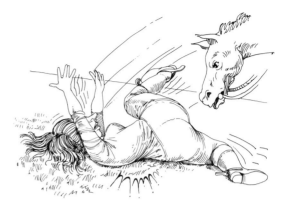

FIG. 4–13. A flexion-rotation injury resulting in a fracture-dislocation of the spine.

FLEXION INJURY
UNSTABLE

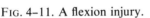

FIG. 4–12. An unstable flexion injury.

FLEXION-ROTATION INJURY
UNSTABLE

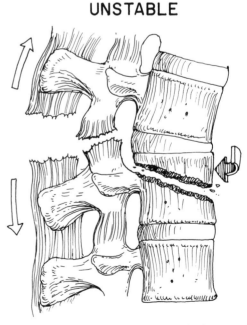

FIG. 4–14. Anatomy of an unstable flexion-rotation injury.

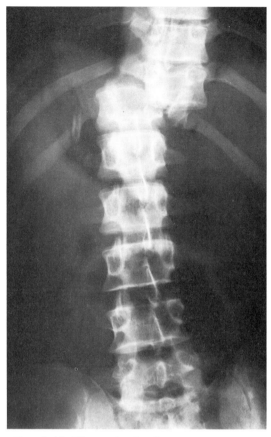

FIG. 4–15. Thoracolumbar fracture-dislocation.

which to compress them. This injury is more common in the cervical spine than in the lumbar spine; it does not occur in the thoracic spine because of the stability offered by the ribs and sternal plate. Pure dislocations such as these are unstable (Fig. 4–12, Table 4–2).

Flexion-Rotation Injury

Flexion-rotation injury results in fracture-dislocations of the spine (Fig. 4–13). The posterior ligamentous complex ruptures, the rotating spine dislocates at the facet joints, and the articulating processes fracture. A slice fracture may also occur in the vertebra below the facet dislocation. In addition, the spinous processes are pulled apart and laterally displaced (Fig. 4–14). This type of injury is consistently associated with paraplegia. In the thoracolumbar area it is very unstable and must be protected, for a partial lesion, or even a cord still untouched, can be converted into a complete lesion (Fig. 4–10, 4–15, Table 4–3).

Hyperextension injuries

In hyperextension injuries (to the cervical spine), the anterior longitudinal ligament and annulus are disrupted and extension-dislocation occurs. The injury becomes stable if the neck is held in flexion. Frequently, roentgenograms taken with the neck in flexion are negative.

Compression Injuries

In compression injuries, the posterior ligamentous complex and the anterior and posterior longitudinal ligaments remain intact, and the spinous processes are not separated. The spine remains stable. However, a fragment that bursts posteriorly may compress the cord and cause tetraplegia in the cervical spine and paraplegia in the lumbar spine.

TABLE 4–3. CRITERIA FOR STABILITY OF THORACOLUMBAR AND LUMBAR SPINE

History of Mechanism of Injury	Stability	Integrity of the Posterior Ligament Complex	Physical Examination		X-ray Findings
			Neurologic Findings (N.F.)	Palpable Spine Defect (P.S.D.)	
Flexion	Stable	Intact	None	None	Wedge vertebrae, minimal separation of the spinal process
Excessive flexion	Unstable	Not intact	N.F.	P.S.D.	Pure vertebral body dislocation. Separation of the spinous process
Flexion-rotation*	Unstable Most unstable of all vertebral injuries.	Not intact	N.F.	P.S.D.	Spinous process separation. Articular process dislocation & fracture. Wedge slice of the lower vertebra
Compression	Stable	Intact	Rare N.F.	None	Burst vertebrae. Spinous processes not separated. Vertebral body is shattered. Fragment may be displaced.
Extension	Stable	Intact. Rare injury. (most common in cervical spine)	N.F.	None	None

*Most common fracture associated with paraplegia

5 Meningomyelocele

DETERMINATION OF LEVEL

Determining the level of neurologic involvement in meningomyelocele is crucial. It permits the evaluation of the following five major functional criteria:

1. Determination of the extent of muscular imbalance around each of the major joints of the lower extremity.
2. Evaluation of the degree and character of any deformity.
3. Assessment of remaining function and the need for bracing or surgery.
4. Evaluation of bladder and bowel function.
5. Baseline analysis for long term follow-up.

Although the defect frequently causes a total loss of innervation below it, this is not always so. In many cases, there will be partial innervation of several levels below the major level of involvement, or partial denervation of several levels above it. It is therefore necessary to determine not only the level which seems to be primarily involved, but also the extent to which other levels may be affected. The level of involvement can be determined through muscle testing, sensory testing, reflex testing, examination of the anus, and evaluation of bladder function.

It is easier to test a newborn infant than a child. In the infant, the skin can be pinched to provide a painful stimulus and the muscle being tested can be palpated for contraction: the muscle will either react (positive indication of muscle function) or will remain inactive (indication of no muscle function). Although it is difficult to grade muscle strength accurately in an infant, it will be evident from palpation and observation whether the muscle is functioning at a minimum of grade three. The infant's muscular function can also be tested by appropriate electrodiagnostic studies such as electromyography and muscle stimulation tests. Children are more difficult to test because they may refuse to respond, forcing the examiner to test many times to obtain an accurate evaluation. In addition, muscle grading is a necessity as soon as it is possible, especially when a child is old enough to cooperate, since the child may lose muscle power or the cord level of involvement may ascend, reducing functional capacity. As a result of such shifting involvement, further evaluation and surgical intervention may be necessary.

Deformities that result from meningomyelocele are usually caused by muscle imbalance. If the muscles around the joint are not working or if all muscles are functioning equally well, deformities seldom develop. It is usually when a muscle is working either unopposed or against a weakened antagonist that a deformity occurs. A mild muscle imbalance acting over a prolonged period of time may produce a deformity. Development of muscle imbalance after birth as a result of the involvement of additional neurologic levels may also lead to deformities. They may also appear as a result of postural problems if braces or splints are incorrectly applied, if the limbs remain constantly in one position until they become fixed, or if the patient is allowed to lie in one position in his crib (in most instances, the hips flex, abduct, and externally rotate, the knees flex, and the feet move into a few degrees of equinus).

Once a fixed deformity has developed, it tends to remain, even if the muscular imbalance disappears. For example, if nerve roots higher than the original lesion become involved, an existing deformity will usually not correct itself even though the previously unopposed muscle has ceased to function.

Evaluate the neurologic or cord level of involvement by motor testing each of the joints of the lower extremity. Then review the information within the broader concepts of neurologic levels to establish the diagnosis (Table 5-1).

The following meningomyelocele examination will evaluate each possible level of involvement from L1-L2 to S2-S3, its functional deficits, and its potential for causing deformity (Fig. 5-1).

TABLE 5-1. MOTOR TESTING FOR NEUROLOGIC LEVEL

Joint	Action	Level
Hip	Flexion	T12, L1, L2, L3
	Extension	S1
	Adduction	L2, L3, L4
	Abduction	L5
Knee	Extension	L2, L3, L4
	Flexion	L5, S1
Ankle	Dorsiflexion (Ankle extension)	L4, L5
	Plantar flexion (Ankle flexion)	S1, S2
	Inversion	L4
	Eversion	S1

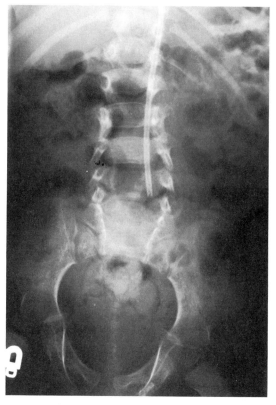

FIG. 5-1. Meningomyelocele.

L1-L2 Neurologic Level (L1 is intact, L2 is not)

Motor Function

HIP

  Flexion: absent
  Extension: absent

  Adduction: absent
  Abduction: absent

No function; there may be some hip flexion from the partial innervation of the iliopsoas (T12, L1, 2, 3).

KNEE

  Extension: absent
  Flexion: absent

No function, no deformity.

FOOT

  Dorsiflexion: absent
  Plantarflexion: absent

  Inversion: absent
  Eversion: absent

No function; if there is any deformity, it may be a result of either the intrauterine position, a loss of function where there was once a muscle imbalance, or a crib position that has produced hip and knee flexion contractures and equinovarus deformity of the foot. The foot normally has a few degrees of equinus when at rest, a position which may become fixed.

Sensory Testing. There is no sensation below the L1 band, which ends approximately one-third of the way down the thigh.

Reflex Testing. None of the deep tendon reflexes of the lower extremity function. Occasionally, reflex activity may occur as a result of the functioning of a portion of the cord below the involved neurologic level (intact reflex arc).

Bladder and Bowel Function. The bladder (S2, S3, S4) is nonfunctioning, the patient is incontinent, the anus is patulous, and the anal wink (S3, S4) is absent. It should be noted that sacral sparing is not uncommon at any level. Lesions which give a pattern of involvement in the sacrally innervated leg muscles but adequate innervation of the sphincter muscles are also common.

L2-L3 Neurologic Level (L2 is intact, L3 is not)

Motor Function

HIP

  Flexion: partial
  Extension: absent

  Adduction: partial
  Abduction: absent

Flexion is considerable, since iliopsoas is almost completely innervated. There is, in addition, a hip flexion deformity because the iliopsoas is unopposed by the major hip extensor, the gluteus maximus (S1, 2). There is a small degree of hip adduction, with a corresponding slight adduction deformity because the adductor group (L2, 3, 4) is partially innervated and is unopposed by the main hip abductor, the gluteus medius (L5, S1).

KNEE

  Extension: partial
  Flexion: absent

The knee is not deformed in spite of the small amount of function of the knee extensor, the quadriceps (L2, 3, 4). There is no significant clinical function.

FOOT. No function, no muscular deformity, except as above.

Sensory Testing. There is no sensation below the L2 band, which ends two-thirds of the way down the thigh.

Reflex Testing. None of the lower extremity reflexes are functioning.

Bladder and Bowel Function. There is no function of the bladder and bowel. The patient cannot urinate in stream when he is quiet; he is only able to dribble urine. A stream may appear if the patient is crying as a result of the tightening of the rectus abdominus muscle and the corresponding increase in intra-abdominal pressure.

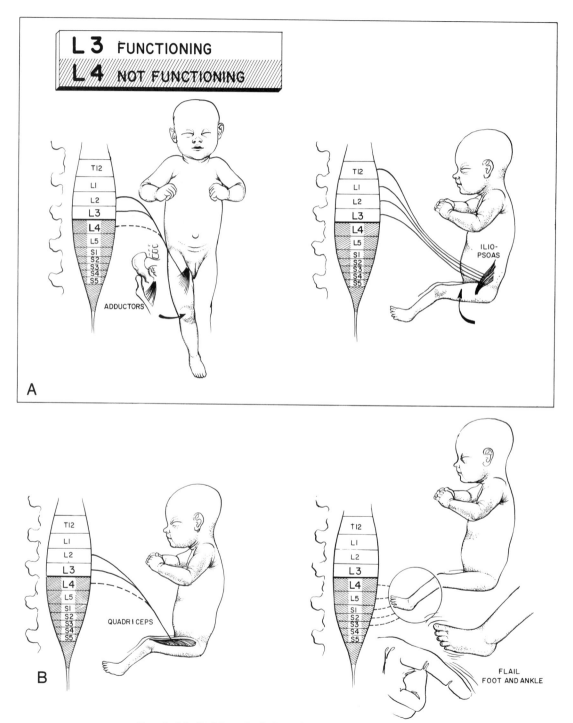

Fig. 5–2A, B. Neurologic Level L3-L4: motor function.

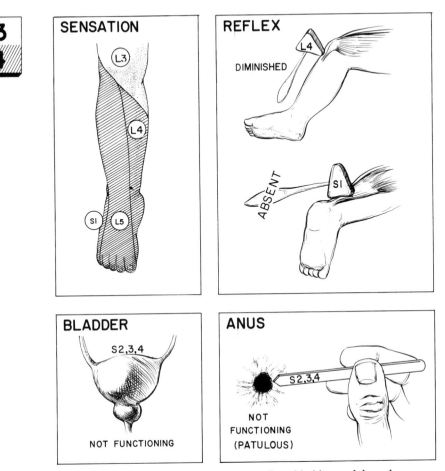

FIG. 5–3. Neurologic level L3-L4: sensation, reflex, bladder and bowel function.

L3-L4 Neurologic Level (L3 is intact, L4 is not)

Motor Function (Fig. 5–2)

HIP

    Flexion: present
    Extension: absent

    Adduction: present
    Abduction: absent

The hip has flexion, adduction, and lateral rotation deformities.

KNEE

    Extension: present
    Flexion: absent

The knee is fixed in extension by the unopposed quadriceps.

FOOT

    Dorsiflexion: absent
    Plantarflexion: absent

    Inversion: absent
    Eversion: absent

There are still no active muscles in the foot.

Sensation Testing (Fig. 5–3). Sensation is normal to the knee. Below the knee, there is no sensation.

Reflex Testing. There may be a slight, but ob-

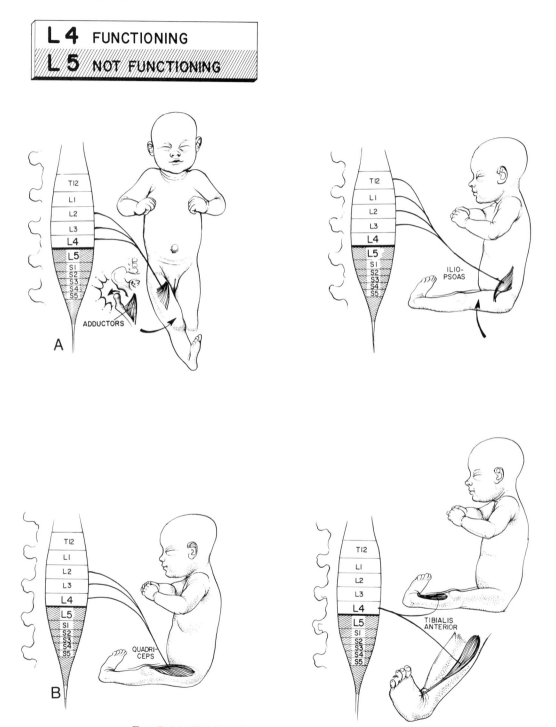

FIG. 5–4A, B. Neurologic level L4-L5: motor function.

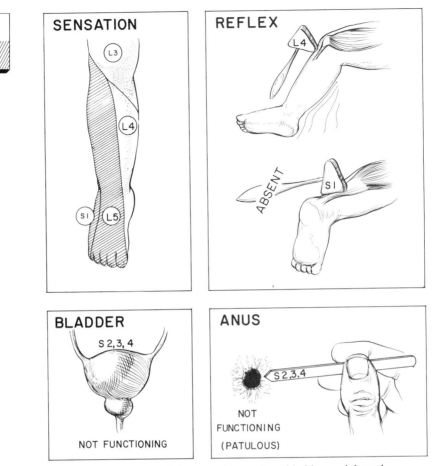

Fig. 5–5. Neurologic level L4-L5: sensation, reflex, bladder and bowel function.

viously diminished, patellar reflex (L2, 3, 4), since the reflex is primarily L4.

Bladder and Bowel Function. No function.

L4-L5 Neurologic Level (L4 is intact, L5 is not)

Motor Function (Fig. 5–4)

HIP

Flexion: present
Extension: absent

Adduction: present
Abduction: absent

The hip has both flexion and adduction deformities, since the iliopsoas and adductor muscles are still unopposed. Such an unop-posed adduction may well result over a time in a dislocated hip and, eventually, a fixed flexion-adduction deformity. For ambulation, full leg bracing will be necessary, including the use of a pelvic band, since the hip is unstable without extension and abduction. Surgery is also a possible solution.

KNEE

Extension: present
Flexion: absent

The knee has an extension deformity as a result of the unopposed action of the quadriceps. The main knee flexors, the medial and lateral hamstrings (L5 and S1), are denervated. An extended knee is relatively stable,

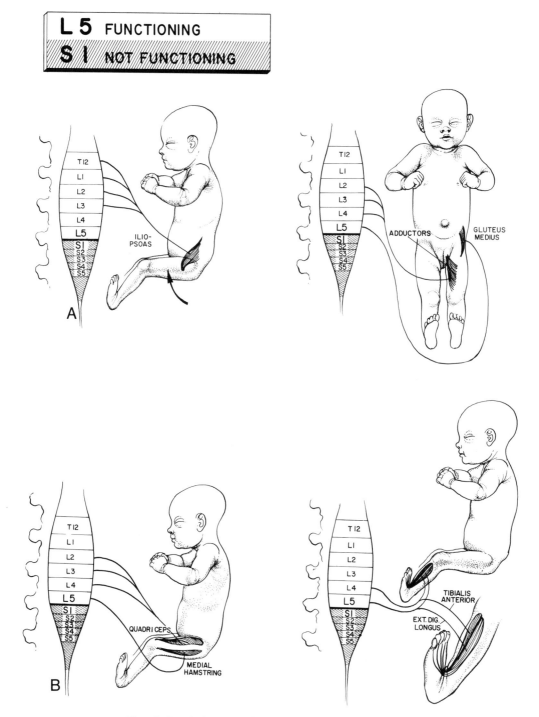

FIG. 5–6A, B. Neurologic level L5-S1: motor function.

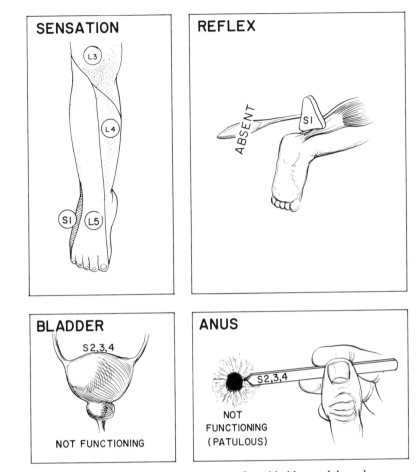

FIG. 5–7. Neurologic level L5-S1: sensation, reflex, bladder and bowel function.

and future bracing is not necessary. However, since the hip must be braced, (unless surgery is performed), the knee is also braced.

FOOT

Dorsiflexion: partial
Plantarflexion: absent

Inversion: partial
Eversion: absent

The only functioning muscle in the foot is the tibialis anterior (L4) because everything else is innervated by L5, S1, S2, and S3. The insertion of the tibialis anterior on the medial side of the foot at the first metatarsal-cuneiform junction causes the foot to be dor-

siflexed and inverted. In this position, the foot is both unbalanced and unstable, and the tibialis anterior may have to be surgically released. The foot is not plantigrade and is without sensation; thus, skin breakdown may occur. Bracing is necessary, but fitting shoes and getting the foot into a brace may be difficult if some correction is not achieved.

Sensory Testing (Fig. 5–5). Sensation extends to the medial side of the tibia and foot. The lateral aspect of the tibia (L5) and the middle and lateral portions of the dorsum of the foot are anesthetic. A pinprick is the most effective way to test infants for sensation; if

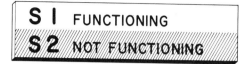

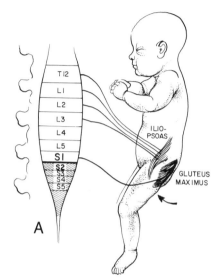

A

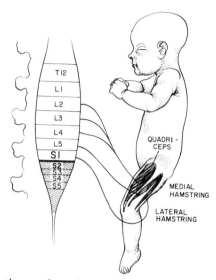

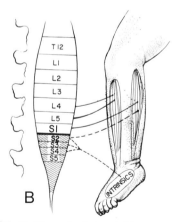

B

Fig. 5–8A, B. Neurologic level S1-S2: motor function.

there is sensation, the child cries or moves the extremity. A triple response to the pinprick (flexion of the hip and knee, dorsiflexion of the foot) should not be confused with motor func-

tion at these joints. Such a general triple reflex response may occur even if the patient is completely paralyzed.

Reflex Testing. The patellar reflex (predominantly L4) functions, whereas the tendon of Achilles reflex (S1) does not. If there is hyperactivity in the tendon of Achilles reflex, a portion of the cord below the original lesion has developed with intact nerve roots, without connection to the rest of the cord. Thus, the S1 ankle reflex arc is intact, and only the inhibitory and controlling factor of the brain is missing.

Bladder and Bowel Function. Neither the bladder nor the bowel function.

L5-S1 Neurologic Level (L5 is intact, S1 is not)

Motor Function (Fig. 5–6)
Hip

    Flexion: present
    Extension: absent

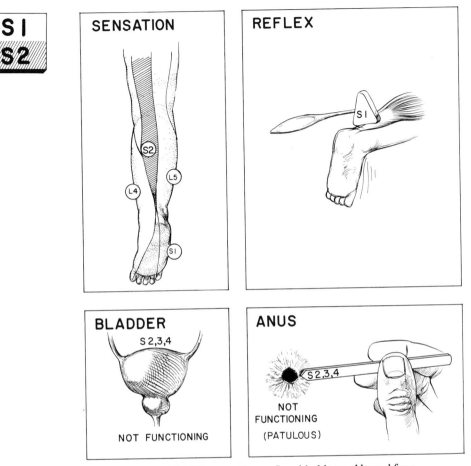

FIG. 5–9. Neurologic level S1–S2: sensation, reflex, bladder and bowel function.

Adduction: present

Abduction: present

There is a flexion deformity of the hip, since the gluteus maximus is not working. There is now a balance between adduction and abduction; however, a minimal adduction deformity may still exist since the gluteus medius, partially supplied by S1, is slightly weak. Because of this partial balance, there is usually no hip dislocation. However, if the gluteus medius is excessively weak, the hip may later sublux. For ambulation, bracing or surgery will be necessary to prevent severe fixed flexion deformity.

KNEE

Extension: present

Flexion: partial

The knee is relatively well balanced, and there are no deformities. The extensors are working; the flexors are functioning in part, with the medial hamstrings (L5) in and the lateral hamstrings (S1) out. Because of this, there may be a slight weakness in flexion. Bracing will be unnecessary.

FOOT

> Dorsiflexion: present
> Plantarflexion: absent
>
> Inversion: present
> Eversion: absent

The dorsiflexors all function. Therefore, the foot will have only a dorsiflexion deformity (calcaneal foot).

Sensory Testing (Fig. 5–7). Sensation is absent on the lateral side and plantar surface of the foot. Elsewhere, it is normal.

Reflex Testing. The tendon of Achilles reflex is still absent.

Bladder and Bowel Function. The bladder and bowel are still nonfunctional.

S1-S2 Neurologic Level (S1 intact, S2 is not)

Motor Function (Fig. 5–8)
HIP

> Flexion: present
> Extension: partial
>
> Adduction: present
> Abduction: present

The hip is almost normal; there may be slight gluteus maximus weakness.

KNEE

> Extension: present
> Flexion: present

The knee is normal and well balanced.

FOOT

> Dorsiflexion: present
> Plantarflexion: partial
>
> Inversion: present
> Eversion: present

The toes of the foot may become clawed, since the intrinsic muscles are still not functioning. In addition, plantar flexion is still weak. Future gait will show weakened or absent toe-off, and the forefoot may be broken on the hindfoot from muscle imbalance (calcaneovalgus of the forefoot). The foot may have a vertical or dislocated talus (convex pes valgus).

Sensory Testing (Fig. 5–9). Sensation is normal except for the posterior strip in the thigh and leg and on the sole of the foot (S4).

Reflex Testing. The tendon of Achilles reflex, although it functions, may be slightly weakened. The reflex is predominantly an S1 reflex with elements of S2.

Bladder and Bowel Function. The bladder and bowel are still not functioning.

S2-S3 Neurologic Level (S2 intact, S3 is not)

Motor Function
HIP. Normal.
KNEE. Normal.
FOOT. The toes of the foot may become clawed in time; there may also be a cavovarus deformity.

Sensory Testing. Sensation is normal.

Reflex Testing. Reflex is normal.

Bladder and Bowel Function. There is often some bladder activity; a portion of the anal wink is present.

MILESTONES OF DEVELOPMENT

Sitting, standing, and walking are three developmental indicators that are useful in determining the future gross motor functional capacity of the patient. Most patients with meningomyelocele experience some delay in reaching these milestones; the amount of delay and degree of difficulty that they encounter provides valuable information as to the course of future rehabilitation.

Sitting. Normally, a child learns to balance himself while sitting at six months of age, and can pull himself to a sitting position at seven to eight months. A child with a lesion above L3 sits late—at approximately ten months—due to muscle weakness around the hips. A child with a high thoracic lesion may have spinal instability, forcing him to balance himself, with the help of his hands, in the tripod position. A spinal fusion stabilizes the spine, freeing the hands for activities of daily living.

Standing. A child is normally able to pull

himself to a standing position at nine to ten months. A child with a thoracic meningomyelocele is unable to do this, no matter what the level of lesion. He should thus be offered bracing for stability; he may still experience some difficulty, however, because braces are both heavy and cumbersome.

Walking. Ambulation normally begins at 12 to 15 months (range; 8 to 18 months). Although almost all children with meningomyelocele have problems with ambulation, independent ambulation with the aid of appliances is possible for those with normal intelligence and involvement in the lumbosacral region. Children are usually more extensively braced than they would be as adults until they reach midadolescence (12 to 15 years). After that time, most patients with lesions higher than S1 will become limited ambulators because of the excessive energy that must be expended as a result of the weight their arms must bear; ambulation with braces and crutches requires as much energy as running at top speed.

UNILATERAL LESIONS

Bifid cords with widely discrepant levels of function are not uncommon. There is a serious possibility that a bony or cartilaginous spur will cause tethering of the cord as the column grows (diastomatomyelia) (Fig. 5–10); any sign of such unilateral loss of function is an indication for a myelogram. Scoliosis, the lateral curvature of the spine, is a significant concomitant problem for those in this group.

HYDROCEPHALUS

From 50 percent to 70 percent of children with meningomyelocele develop hydrocephalus, an abnormal increase in the ventricular size, resulting in enlargement of the head and abnormal prominence of the forehead. Hydrocephalus usually develops secondary to Arnold-Chiari malformation (caudal displace-

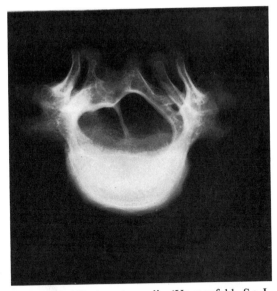

Fig. 5–10. Diastomatomyelia (Hoppenfeld, S.: J. Bone Joint Surg., *493*:276, 1967).

ment of the brain stem). If it is left unattended, it can lead to spasticity that may further decrease already compromised muscle function on either marginally or normally innervated muscles. If hydrocephalus is treated early, ventricular size, and thereby head circumference, can be maintained within normal limits. The usual method of therapy is with a shunt and appropriate revisions, if necessary. The shunt is a tube that drains excess spinal fluid from the ventricles of the brain to the peritoneal cavity or heart.

EXAMINATION OF THE UPPER EXTREMITY

Although the great majority of meningomyelocele lesions occur in the lumbosacral region, higher lesions affecting the function of the upper extremity may occur in association with these lower lesions, necessitating a complete neurologic evaluation of the upper extremity. Hydromyelia (enlargement of the central canal of the spinal cord) and syrin-

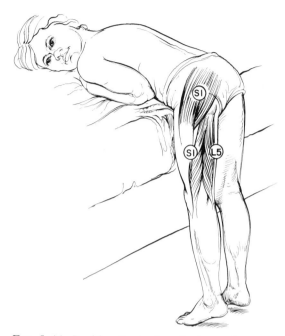

FIG. 5–11. Position for testing the hamstring and gluteus maximus muscles.

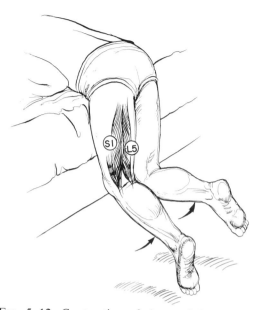

FIG. 5–12. Contraction of the medial hamstring muscle indicates integrity of L5 neurologic level; contraction of the lateral hamstring muscle indicates integrity of S1 neurologic level.

gomyelia (liquid filling abnormal cavities in the substance of the spinal cord) of the cervical cord may also occur in association with meningomyelocele of the lumbar and sacral regions. Both these pathologies are progressive and require careful motor and sensory testing of the upper extremity with provisions for follow-up care. To patients with meningomyelocele, the upper extremities are particularly important because of their use in crutch walking.

SUGGESTIONS FOR EXAMINATION OF THE PATIENT WITH MENINGOMYELOCELE

1. Do not mistake the withdrawal response for voluntary control of motor power. Even though a pin-prick stimulus may cause withdrawal at three joints—hip flexion, knee flex-

ion, and ankle dorsiflexion (the triple response)—the infant does not necessarily feel the noxious stimulus. It is necessary to watch the child for signs of crying and changes in facial expression to determine whether there exists a *central recognition* of pain.

2. To muscle test the hamstrings, position the patient face down on the edge of the examining table, so that his hips and lower extremities hang freely (Fig. 5–11). Stabilize him. Then determine whether he can flex his knees. If the knee flexes, it is working against gravity and is acting with at least grade three strength (Fig. 5–12). During testing, palpate medially to determine activity of the semimembranosus and semitendinosus (L5) and laterally for the biceps femoris (S1).

3. To muscle test the gluteus maximus, continue to hold the patient in the same position and have him extend his hips, indicating

gluteus maximus activity (S1) (Fig. 5–13).

4. It is by far easier to evaluate function in young children by playing with them than by conducting a formal examination.

5. Make certain that the patient is warm and comfortable during the examination.

6. Have the nursing staff record their observations of any spontaneous movements of the patient's extremities.

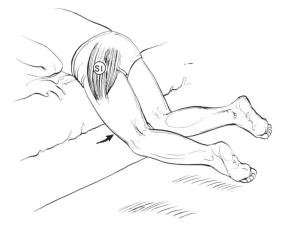

FIG. 5–13. Contraction of the gluteus maximus indicates integrity of S1 neurologic level.

REFERENCES

Abbott, K.H., and Retter, R: Protrusions of thoracic intervertebral disks, Neurology, *6*: 1, 1955.

Abramson, A.S.: Bone disturbances in injuries to the spinal cord and cauda equina, Bone Joint Surg., *30-A*: 982, 1948.

– – –: Principles of bracing in the rehabilitation of the paraplegic, Bull. Hosp. Joint Dis., *X*: 175, 1949.

– – –: Changing concepts in the management of spasticity, p. 205-228 in French, J.D. Ed. Conference in basic research in paraplegia, Thomas 1962.

– – –: Modern concepts of management of the patient with spinal cord injury, Arch. Phys. Med. Rehabil., *48*: 113, 1967.

– – –: Advances in the management of the neurogenic bladder, Arch. Phys. Med., *52*: 143, 1971.

– – –: Management of the neurogenic bladder in perspective. Arch. Phys. Med. Rehabil., *57*: 197, 1976.

Abramson, A.S. and Delagi, E.F.: Influence of weight bearing and muscle contraction on disuse osteoporosis, Arch. Phys. Med. Rehabil., *42*: 147, 1961.

Aegerter, E., Kirkpatrick, J.A. Jr.: Orthopaedic Diseases: Physiology, Pathology, Radiology, ed. 3, Philadelphia, Saunders, 1968.

Alexander, M.A., Bunch, W.H. Ebbesson, S.O. Can experimental dorsal rhizotomy produce scoliolis? J. Bone Joint Surg. *54*: 1509-1513: 1972.

American Academy of Orthopaedic Surgeons: Symposium on Myelomeningocele, St. Louis, Mosby, 1972.

Apley, A.G.: Fractures of the spine, Ann. R. Coll. Surg., *46*: 210, 1970.

– – –: A System of Orthopaedics and Fractures, ed. 4, London, Butterworth, 1973.

Arseni, C, and Nash, R.: Thoracic intervertebral disc protrusion. J. Neurosurg., *17*: 418, 1960.

Bailey, R.W., and Badgley, C.E.: Stabilization of the cervical spine by anterior fusion, J. Bone Joint Surg., *42A*: 565, 1960.

Bannister, R.: Brain's Clinical Neurology, ed. 4, London, Oxford, 1973.

Barr, M.L.: The Human Nervous System: An Anatomical Viewpoint, ed. 2, Hagerstown, Harper & Row, 1974.

Basmajian, J.V.: Muscles Alive, ed. 3, Baltimore, Williams & Wilkins, 1974.

Bateman, J.E.: Trauma to Nerves in Limbs, Philadelphia, Saunders, 1962.

Bauer, D.D.: Lumbar Discography and Low Back Pain, Springfield, Thomas, 1960.

Beetham, W.P. Jr., Polley, H.F., Slocumb, C.H., Weaver, W.F.: Physical Examination of the Joints, Philadelphia, Saunders, 1965.

Bender, M.B.: Approach to diagnosis in modern neurology, Mt. Sinai J. Med. N.Y. *33*: 201, 1966.

Benson, M.K.D., and Byrnes, D.P.: The clinical syndromes and surgical treatment of thoracic intervertebral disc prolapse, J. Bone Joint Surg. *57B*: 471, 1975.

Bernes, S.H.: Spinal Cord Injury: Rehabilitation Costs and Results in 31 Successive Cases Including a Follow-Up Study, (Rehabilitation Monograph). New York Institute of Physical Medicine & Rehabilitation, New York University-Bellevue Hospital, 1957.

Bickerstaff, E.R,: Neurologic Examination in Clinical Practice, ed. 3, Oxford, Blackwell, 1973.

Bowens, P.: Electrodiagnosis and electrotherapy in peripheral nerve lesions, Proc. R. Soc. Med., *34*: 459, 1941.

Bowsher, D.: Introduction to the Anatomy and Physiology of the Nervous System, ed. 3, Oxford, Blackwell, 1975.

Boyes, J.H.: Bunnell's Surgery of the Hand, ed. 3, Philadelphia, Lippincott, 1970.

Bristow, R.: Discussion on injuries to peripheral nerves, Proc. R. Soc. Med., *34*: 513, 1941.

Brock, S., and Kreiger, H.P.: The Basis of Clinical Neurology, ed. 4, Baltimore, Williams & Wilkins, 1893.

Brown-Sequard, C.E.: Course of Lectures on Physiology and Pathology of CNS Delivered at Royal College of Surgeons, England 1858, Collins, Philadelphia, 1860.

Caafoord, C., Hiertonn, T., Lindblom, K., and Olsson S.E.: Spinal cord compression caused by a protruded thoracic disc. Report of a case treated with antero-lateral fenestration of the disc. Acta Ortho. Scand., ·*28*: 103, 1958.

Capener, N.: The evolution of lateral rhacotomy, J. Bone Joint Surg. *36-B*: 173, 1954.

Carson, J., Gumper, J., and Jefferson, A.: Diagnosis and treatment of thoracic intervertebral disc protrusions, J. Neur. Neurosurg. Psychiatry, *34*: 68-77, 1971.

Chesterman, P.J.: Spastic paraplegia caused by sequestrated thoracic intervertebral disc, Pro. R. Soc. Med., *57*: 87, 1964.

Chusid, Joseph, G., McDonald, Joseph J: Correlative Neuroanatomy and Functional Neurology, Los Altos, Cal., Lange, 1967.

Clark, K.: Peripheral nerve injury associated with fractures, Postgrad. Med., *27*: 476, 1960.

Clark, E.: The Human Brain and Spinal Cord: a Historical Study Illustrated by Writing From Antiquity, Berkeley, University of California, 1968.

Cloward, R.B.: Treatment of acute fractures and fracture-dislocations of the cervical spine by vertical-body fusion, J. Neurosurg., *18*: 201, 1961.

– – –: Surgical treatment of dislocations and compression fractures of the cervical spine by the anterior approach, Proc. Ann. Clin. Spinal Cord Injury Conf., 11, Veterans Admin., Washington, 1970.

Crenshaw, A.H.: Campbell's Operative Orthopaedics, ed. 5, St. Louis, Mosby, 1971.

Crosby, E., Humphrey, T., Lauer, E.W.: Correlative Anatomy of the Nervous System, New York, Macmillan, 1962.

Daniels, L., Williams, M., Worthingham, C.: Muscle Testing – Techniques of Manual Examination, ed. 2, Saunders, Philadelphia, 1946.

DeJong, Russel, N.: The Neurologic Examination, ed. 3, New York, Harper & Row, 1967.

Delagi, E., Perrotto, A., Iazzetti, J., Morrison, D.: An Anatomic Guide for the Electromyographer, Springfield, Thomas, 1975.

Dodson, W.E., Landau, W.: Motor Neuron loss due to aortic clamping in repair of coarctation, Neurology *23 (5)*: 539, 1973.

Dommisse, G.F.: The blood supply of the spinal cord, J. Bone Joint Surg. *56B*: 225, 1974.

Draper, I.T.: Lecture Notes on Neurology, ed. 4, Oxford, Blackwell, 1974.

Dunkerley, G.B.: A Basic Atlas of the Human Nervous System. Davis, Philadelphia, 1975.

Elliot, H.: Textbook of Neuroanatomy, ed. 2, Philadelphia, Lippincott, 1969.

Everett, N.B., Bodemier, C.W., Rieke, W.O.: Functional Neuroanatomy including an Atlas of the Brain Stem, ed. 5, Philadelphia, Lea & Febiger, 1965.

Favill, J.: Outline of the Spinal Nerves, Springfield, Thomas, 1946.

Ferguson, A.B.: Orthopaedic Surgery in Infancy and Childhood, ed. 3, Baltimore, Williams & Wilkins, 1968.

Fielding, J.W.: Cineroentgenography of the normal cervical spine, J. Bone Joint Surg., *39A*: 1280, 1957.

Fisher, R.G.: Protrusions of thoracic disc; the factor of herniation through the dura mater, J. Neurosurg., *22*: 591, 1965.

Globus, J.H.: Neuroanatomy; a guide for the study of the form and internal structure of the brain and spinal cord, ed. 6, Baltimore, Wood, 1934.

Guttmann, L: Surgical aspects of the treatment of traumatic paraplegia, J. Bone Joint Surg., *31B*: 399, 1949.

– – –: Early management of the paraplegic in Symposium on Spinal Injuries, J. R. Col. Surg., 1963.

– – –: Spinal Cord Injuries; Comprehensive Management and Research, Oxford, Blackwell, 1973.

Guyton, A.C.: Structure and Function of the Nervous System, Philadelphia, Saunders, 1972.

Haley, J.C., Perry, J.H.: Protrusions of intervertebral discs. Study of their distribution, characteristics and effects on the nervous system, Am. J. Surg., 80: 394, 1950.

Hardy, A.G., Rossier, A.B.: Spinal Cord Injuries, Orthopaedic and Neurological Aspects, Stuttgart, Thieme, 1975.

Harrington, P.: Spinal fusion in the treatment of idiopathic adolescent scoliosis, J. Tenn. Med. Assoc., 56: 470, 1963.

Hausman, L.: Illustrations of the Nervous System: Atlas III, Springfield, Thomas, 1961.

Hawk, W.A.: Spinal compression caused by ecchondrosis of the intervertebral fibrocartilage; with a review of the recent literature, Brain, 59: 204, 1936.

Haymaker, W., Woodhall, B., Peripheral Nerve Injuries, Philadelphia, Saunders, 1953.

Helfet, A.J.: Disorders of the Knee, Philadelphia, Lippincott, 1974.

Hendry, A.: The treatment of residual paralysis after brachial plexus injuries, J. Bone Joint Surg., *31B*: 42, 1949.

Henry, A.K: Extensile Exposure, ed. 2, Baltimore, Williams and Wilkins, 1959.

Holdsworth, F.W.: Fractures, dislocations, and fracture-dislocations of the spine, J. Bone Joint Surg., *45B*: 6, 1963.

– – –: Fractures, dislocations and fracture-dislocations of the spine, J.Bone Joint Surg., 52A: 1534-1551, 1970.

Holdsworth, F.W., Hardy, A.: Early treatment of paraplegia from fractures of the thoracolumbar spine, J. Bone Joint Surg., 35B: 540, 1953.

Hollinshead, W.H.: Anatomy for Surgeons. The Back and Limbs, vol. 3, New York, Hoeber, 1958.

Holmes, R.L. and Sharp, J.A.: The Human Nervous System: a Devlopmental Approach, London, Churchill 1969.

Hoppenfeld, S.: Congenital kyphosis in myelomeningocele, J. Bone Joint Surg., *49B*: 1967.

– – –: Physical Examination of the Spine and Extremities, New York, Appleton Century Croft, 1976.

– – –: Scoliosis, Philadelphia, Lippincott, 1967.

House, E.L., Pansky, B.: A Functional Approach to Neuroanatomy, New York, McGraw-Hill, 1960.

Howorth, B., Petrie, J.G.: Injuries of the Spine, Baltimore, Williams & Wilkins, 1964.

Hulme, A.: The surgical approach to thoracic intervertebral disc protrusions, J. Neuro. Neurosurg. Psychiatry, 23: 133, 1960.

Hussey, R.W., Stauffer, E.S.: Spinal cord injury; requirements for ambulation, Arch. Phys. Med., 54: 544, 1973.

Kaplan, E.B.: The surgical and anatomic significance of the mammillary tubercle of the last thoracic vertebra, Surgery, 17: 78, 1945.

– – –(translator): Duchenne, G.W.: Physiology of Motion, Philadelphia, Saunders, 1959.

Keim, H.A., Hilal, S.D.: Spinal angiography in scliosis patients, J. Bone Joint Surg., 53A: 904, 1971.

Kelikian, H.: Hallux Valgus, Allied Deformities of the Forefoot and Metatarsalgia, Philadelphia, Saunders, 1965.

Kilfoyle, R.M., Foley, J.J., Norton, P.L.: Spine and pelvic · deformity in childhood and adolescent paraplegia. A study of 104 cases, J. Bone Joint Surg., 47A: 659, 1965.

Kostiuk, P.G., Skibo, G.G.: Structural characteristics of the connections of the medial descending systems with the neurons of the spinal cord., Neirofiziologiia 4(6): 579, 1972.

Krieg, W.J.: Functional Neuroanatomy, ed. 3, Evanston, Ill., Brain Books, 1966.

Kroll, F.W., Reiss, E.: Der thorakale Bandscheibenprolaps, Dtsch. Med. Wochenschr., 76: 600, 1951.

Kuntz, A.: A Textbook of Neuroanatomy, ed. 5, Philadelphia, Lea & Febiger, 1950.

Larsell, O.: Anatomy of Nervous System, ed. 2, New York, Appleton-Century-Crofts, 1951.

Lees, F.: The Diagnosis and Treatment of Diseases Affecting the Nervous System, London, Staples Press, 1970.

Leffert, R.D.: Brachial-plexus injuries, New Eng. J. Med., 291(20): 1059, 1974.

Lewin, P.: The Foot and Ankle, Philadelphia, Lea & Febiger, 1958.

Logue, V.: Thoracic intervertebral disc prolapse with spinal cord compression, J. Neur., Neurosurg. Psychiatry, 15: 227, 1952.

Love, J.G., Keifer, E.J.: Root pain and paraplegia due to protrusions of thoracic intervertebral disks, J. Neurosurg., 7: 62, 1950.

Love, J.G., Schorn, V.G: Thoracic disc protrusions, JAMA, 191: 627, 1965.

Lyons, W.R., Woodhall, B.: Atlas of peripheral nerve injuries, Philadelphia, Saunders, 1949.

McBride, E.D.: Disability Evaluation, ed. 5, Philadelphia, Lippincott, 1953.

Mac Nab, I.: Acceleration of injuries of cervical spine, J. Bone Joint Surg., *46A*: 1797, 1964.

Malamud, N., Hirano, A.: Atlas of Neuropathology, Berkeley, Univ. California Press, 1974.

Manter, J.T., Gatz, J.: Essentials of Clinical Neuroanatomy and Neurophysiology, ed. 5, Philadelphia, Davis, 1975.

Mathews, W.: Diseases of the Nervous System, ed. 2, Oxford, Blackwell, 1975.

Medical & Technical Summaries Inc.: Neuroanatomy, 1959-60 ed., Washington, Sigma Press, 1959.

Menard, V.: Etude Pratique sur le Mal du Pott, Paris, Masson, 1900.

Mercer, W., Duthie, R.B.: Orthopaedic Surgery, London, Arnold, 1964.

Mettler, F.A.: Neuroanatomy, ed. 2, St. Louis, Mosby, 1948.

Michaelis, L.S.: Orthopaedic Surgery of the Limbs in Paraplegia, Berlin, Springer, 1964.

Middleton, G.S., Teacher, J.H.: Injury of the spinal cord due to rupture of an intervertebral disc during muscular effort, Glasgow Med. J., *76*: 1-6, 1911.

Mitchell, G.A.G.: Essentials of Neuroanatomy, Edinborough, Livingstone, 1971.

Mixter, W.J., Barr, J.S.: Rupture of the intervertebral disc with involvement of the spinal canal. New Eng. J. Med., *211*: 210, 1934.

Morris, J.M., Lucas, D.B., Bresler, B.: Role of the trunk in stability of the spine, J. Bone Joint Surg., *43A*: 327, 1961.

Muller, R.: Protrusions of thoracic intervertebral disks with compression of the spinal cord, Acta Med. Scandin., *139*: 99, 1951.

Nachemson, A.: The lumbar spine, an orthopaedic challenge, Spine 1: 69, 1976.

Nachemson, A., Morris, J.: In vivo measurement of intradiscal pressure, J. Bone Joint Surg., *46A*: 1077, 1964.

Naffziger, H.C.: The neurological aspects of injuries to the spine, J. Bone Joint Surg., *20*: 444, 1938.

Netter, F.H.: The Ciba Collection of Medical Illustrations, Ciba Pharmaceutical Products, 1953.

Newman, P.H.: The etiology of spondylolisthesis, J. Bone Joint Surgery, *45B*: 1963.

Nicoll, E.A.: Fractures of the dorsolumbar spine, J. Bone Joint Surg., *31B*: 376, 1949.

Olsson, O.: Fractures of the upper thoracic and cervical vertebral bodies, Acta Chir. Scand., *102*: 87, 1951.

Peck, F.C.: A calcified thoracic intervertebral disk with herniation and spinal cord compression in a child, J. Neurosurg., *14*: 105, 1957.

Peele, T.L.: The Neuroanatomic Basis for Clinical Neurology, ed. 2, New York, Blakiston, 1961.

Perlman, S.G.: Spinal cord injury; a review of experimental implications for clinical prognosis and treatment, Arch. Phys. Med. Rehab., *55*: 81, 1974.

Perot, P.L, Jr., Munro, D.D.: Transthoracic removal of thoracic disc, J. Neurosurg., *31*: 452, 1969.

Perry, C.B.W.: The management of injuries to the brachial plexus, Proc. R. Soc. Med., *67(6)*: 488, 1974.

Perry, C., Nickel, V.L.: Total cervical fusion for neck paralysis, J. Bone Joint Surg., *41-A*: 37, 1959.

Petrie, J.G.: Flexion injuries of the cervical spine, J. Bone Joint Surg., *46-A*: 1800, 1964.

Pool, J.L.: The Neurosurgical Treatment of Traumatic Paraplegia, Springfield, Thomas, 1951.

Quiring, D.P., Warfel, J.H.: The Extremities, Philadelphia, Lea & Febiger, 1967.

Ranney, A.L.: The applied anatomy of the nervous system, being a study of this portion of the human body from a standpoint of its general interest and practical utility, designed for use as a textbook and a work of reference, New York, Appleton, 1881.

Ransohoff, J., Spencer, F., Siew, F., Gage, L.: Transthoracic removal of thoracic disc, J. Neurosurg., *31*: 459, 1969.

Ranson, S.W., Clark, S.L.: The Anatomy of the Nervous System: Its Development and Function, ed. 10, Philadelphia, Saunders, 1959.

Reeves, D.L., Brown, H.A.: Thoracic intervertebral disc protrusion with spinal cord compression, J. Neurosurg., *28*: 14, 1968.

Roaf, R.: A study of the mechanics of spinal injuries., J. Bone Joint Surg., *42-B*: 810, 1960.

Salter, R.B.: Textbook of Disorders and Injuries of the Musculoskeletal System, Baltimore, Williams & Wilkins, 1970.

Sandiffer, P.H.: Neurology in Orthopaedics, London, Butterworth, 1967.

Santee, H.E.: Anatomy of Brain and Spinal Cord, ed. 3, Chicago, Colegrove, 1903.

Schneider, R.C.: Surgical indications and contraindications in spine and spinal cord trauma, Clin. Neurosurg., 8: 157, 1962.

Schultz, R.J.: The Language of Fractures, Williams & Wilkins, Baltimore, 1972.

Seddon, H.J., ed: Peripheral Nerve Injuries, Medical Research Council Spec. Report Series No. 282, London, H.M. Stationery Office, 1954.

Seddon, H.J.: Surgery of nerve injuries, Practitioner, *184*: 181, 1960.

Sharrard, W.J.W.: The distribution of permanent paralysis in the lower limb in poliomyelitis; A clinical and pathological study, J. Bone Joint Surg., *37-B*: 540, 1955.

— — —: Muscle paralysis in poliomyelitis, Br. J. Surg., *44*: 471, 1957.

— — —: Poliomyelitis and the anatomy of the motor cell columns in the spinal cord, Extrait du VII Symposium, Oxford 17-20: 241-245, 1961.

— — —: Posterior iliopsoas transplantation in the treatment of paralytic dislocation of the hip, J. Bone Joint Surg., *46-B*: 1964.

— — —: The segmental innervation of the lower limb muscles in man, An. R. Col. Surg. (Eng.), *35*: 106, 1964.

— — —: Paediatric Orthopaedics and Fractures, Oxford, Blackwell, 1971.

— — —: Spina Bifida, A Symposium on Paralysis

Shore, N.A.: Occlusal Equilibration and Temporomandibular Joint Dysfunction, ed. 2, Philadelphia, Lippincott, 1976.

Sidman, R.L., Sideman, M.: Neuranatomy: A Programmed Text, Boston, Little, Brown, 1965.

Smith, C.G.: Basic Neuroanatomy, ed. 2, Toronto, Univ. Toronto Press, 1971.

Southwick, W.O., Robinson, R.A.: Surgical approaches to the vertebral bodies in the cervical and lumbar regions, J. Bone Joint Surg., *39-A*: 631, 1957.

Spinner, M.: Injuries to the Major Branches of Peripheral Nerves of the Forearm, Philadelphia, Saunders, 1972.

Spofford, W.R.: Neuroanatomy, London, Oxford Univ. Press, 1942.

Stauffer, E.S.: Orthopaedic care of fracture dislocations of the cervical spine, Proc. Ann. Veterans Admin. Clin. Spinal Cord Injury Conf., Washington, Veterans Admin., 1970.

Steegmann, A.J.: Examination of the Nervous System, Chicago, Year Book, 1956.

Steindler, A.: Kinesiology of the Human Body, Springfield, Thomas, 1955.

Suttong, N.G.: Injuries of the Spinal Cord, The Management of Paraplegia and Tetraplegia, London, Butterworth, 1973.

Svien, H.J., Karaviti, A.L.: Multiple protrusions of the intervertebral disks in the upper thoracic region, Proc. Mayo Clinic, *29*: 375-378, 1954.

Swan, J.: A Demonstration of the Nerves of the Human Body, London, Longman, 1834.

Tachdjian, M.O.: Pediatric Orthopaedics, Vol: 1, 2, Philadelphia, Saunders, 1972.

Taiushey, K.G.: Changes in the spinal cord following its complete sectioning at the so-called critical levels, Arch. Anat. Histol. Embryol. (Strasb), 86, 1971.

Thomson, J.L.G.: Meylography in dorsal disc protrusion, Acta Radio. [Diagn.] (Stockh.), *5*: 1140, 1966.

Truex, R.C., Carpenter, M.B.: Human Neuroanatomy, ed. 5, Baltimore, Williams & Wilkins' 1969.

Turek, S.L.: Orthopaedics: Principles and Their Application, ed. 2, Philadelphia, Lippincott, 1967.

Watson-Jones, R.: Primary nerve lesions in injuries of the elbow and wrist, J. Bone Joint Surg., *12*: 121, 1930.

— — —: Fractures and Joint Injuries, ed. 4, vol. 2, Baltimore, Williams & Wilkins, 1955.

Weiner, H.L., Levitt, L.P.: Neurology for the House Officer, New York, Med. Com., 1973, 1974.

Whitesides, T.E., Kelley, R., Howland, S.C.: The treatment of lumbodorsal fracture-dislocations (abstr), J. Bone Joint Surg., *52-A*: 1267, 1970.

Winter, R.B., Moe, J.H., Wang, J.F.: Congenital kyphosis. Its natural history and treatment as observed in a study of 130 patients, J. Bone Joint Surg., *55-A*: 223, 1973.

Wyke, B.D.: Principles of General Neurology, New York, Elsevier, 1969.

Zachs, S.I.: Atlas of Neuropathology, New York, Harper & Row, 1971.

Index

Numbers in *italics* indicate a figure.

Abduction, hip, *56*
  shoulder, in tetraplegia, level C5, 80
Abductors, finger, 23, *24*, 25
  shoulder, *8, 9*
Ache. *See* Pain
Achilles tendon reflex, *58*, 65
  herniated lumbar disc, 66, *68–70*
  herniated thoracic disc, 101
  memory aid, 63
  meningomyelocele, level L5-S1, *115*, 118
  spinal cord damage, levels L1-S1, 94–95
  testing, 61, 63, *63*
Adductor brevis, longus and magnus, *50*
Adductors, meningomyelocele, level L3-L4, *110*
  level L4-L5, *112*
  level L5-S1, *114*
  spinal cord lesions, levels L2-L4, 94
Ambulation, meningomyelocele, 113
  spinal cord lesions, 84, 90
  prognostication, 98
  See also Wheelchair
Anal wink, 64, 99, 118
Ankle, extension, *54, 55*
  flexion, *60*
Annulus fibrosus, cervical, *30*
  lumbar, *67*
Antebrachial cutaneous nerve, 23
Arms, pain, and herniated disc, 29
  and meningomyelocele, 119
  spinal cord lesion, level C6, 81
    level C8, 83
    level T1, 83–84
  testing, memory aid, level C6, *17*
    level C8, *23*
    neurologic level C5, 7–12, *8–13*
    neurologic level C6, 13–17, *13–17*
    neurologic level C7, 17–21, *18–21*

Arms, testing—(*Continued*)
    neurologic level C8, 21–23, *22–23*
  See also Extremity, upper
Atlas, cervical spine, 1
Axillary nerve, 7–8, *8*, 12, *13*

Babinski's sign, 95, *95*
Backache. *See* Pain
Beevor's sign, 45, *45*, 93, 100
Biceps brachii, *10*
  testing, 11–12, *12*
  herniated disc, *32–36*
  spinal cord damage, level C5, 80
    level C6, 81
Biceps tendon reflex, *8*
  herniated disc, *32–36*
  testing, 12, *12*, 13, 27
    memory aid, *12*
  tetraplegia, *78–84*
  spinal cord lesion, level C5, 80
    level C6, 82
    level C7, 82
Bladder and bowel function, herniated thoracic disc, 101
  meningomyelocele, levels L1-L2, L2-L3, 109
    level L3-L4, *111*, 113
    level L4-L5, *113*, 116
    level L5-S1, *115*, 118
    level S1-S2, *117*, 118
    level S2-S3, 118
  spinal cord damage, levels L1-S1, 94–95
  prognostication, 98–100
Brachialis, *10*
Brachial-cutaneous nerve, sensation test, 25
Brachioradialis reflex, with herniated discs, *32–36*
  spinal cord damage, 82
  testing, 13, *14, 16*, 27
  tetraplegia, *78–84*
Bulbocavernosus reflex, 99, *100*

Calf muscles, level affecting, 74

Carotid tuberosity, 7
Cauda equina, 45, 93
  and nerve roots, 66
  sacral sparing, *97*, 97
  spinal cord lesions, 94–105
Cells, anterior horn, in poliomyelitis, 72, *73*
Cervical discs. *See* Disc, cervical
Cervical nerves. *See* Nerve roots, cervical
Cervical spine. *See* Spine, cervical
Cervical vertebrae. *See* Vertebrae
Compression fracture, of neck, 86, *87, 88*
Compression test, of osteoarthritis, 42, *43*
Cord, spinal. *See* Spinal Cord
Cremasteric reflex, 96, *96*
Crutch, arm muscle use, 19
  spinal cord lesions, levels C3-T1, 90–91

D.A.B., dorsal interossei, 23–25
Deformity in meningomyelocele, 108
  level L3-L4, 111
  level L4-L5, 113
  level L5-S1, 117–118
  level S1-S2, 118
  level S2-S3, 118
Deltoid, with herniated discs, *32–36*
  testing, 7–9, *8–9*
  in tetraplegia, *78–84*
  with spinal cord damage, 80
Dermatomes, definition, 1
  diagram, 2
  of feet, 65
  herpes zoster, 71
  of lower extremity, 49, *51*
  level L4, 56
  level L4-S1, *68–70*
  level L5, 59
  levels S2, 3, 4, 5, *64*
  of trunk, 94
  upper extremity, 27
Development milestones, 118–119

Diastomatomyelia, 119, *119*
Disc, cervical, 1
  herniated, 28–40, *28*
    anatomic basis, *30*
    cord damage, 91
    electromyogram, 37
    myelogram, *37*
    neurologic levels, *32–36*
      table, 38
    tests for location, 31–37, *32–36*
    Valsalva test, 39
  lumbar, herniated, 66–68, *67–71*
    myelogram, *71*
    table, 66
  thoracic, herniated, 100–101
Dislocation, of spine, 102, 104
  cervical, 85–90, *88–90*
Distraction test, of osteoarthritis, 42, *43*
Dorsal interossei (D.A.B.), testing, 23–25, *24*

Elbow, flexion and extension, 10–12, *10–12*
  with spinal cord damage, level C6, 81
Electromyogram, (EMG), herniated disc, 37
  table, 38, 66
Examination, meningomyelocele, 120
  See also Testing
Extension lag, of knee, *48*, 49
Extensor carpi radialis, 13, *14–15*
Extensor carpi ulnaris, 13, *14–15*
Extensor digiti minimi, 21
Extensor digitorum, *20*, 21
  brevis, *55*, 57, 59
  longus, *54, 55*
    meningomyelocele, level L5-S1, *114*
    testing, 57, 59, 74
    for herniated discs, *68–70*
Extensor hallucis longus, *54, 55,* 74
  and herniated disc, table, 66
  testing, 57
Extensor indicis proprius, 21
Extensors, toe, memory aid, *55*
Extremity, lower, nerve root lesions, 45–74
  upper, sensory summary, *27*
  neurologic levels, *28*
  testing, scheme of, 25–28
  nerve root lesions, 7–43
  See also Arms, Legs, Fingers, Toes, Hand, Foot, etc.

Facet joint, capsule, 101, *101*
  dislocations, 88–90, *88–90*

Femoral nerve, 47, 74
Fingers, abduction, testing, 23–25, *23–25*
  adduction, testing, *24,* 25, *26*
  extensors, *20,* 21
    with herniated discs, *32–36*
    with spinal cord damage, 82
    in tetraplegia, *78–84*
  flexors, 21
    muscle test, 21–23, *20–23*
    with herniated disc, *32–36*
    sensation testing, 21, 23
    in spinal cord lesion, 83
Flaccidity, of muscle, 97–98
Flexor carpi radialis, 17, 20, *19*
Flexor carpi ulnaris, 17, *19,* 20
Flexor digitorum, 21–23, *20, 22,* 74
Flexor hallucis, 74
Foot, dermatome, 59, *63*
  dorsiflexion, *54, 55*
  eversion, *58*
  flail, *110*
    meningomyelocele, levels L1-L2, L2-L3, 109
    level L3-L4, *110,* 111
    level L4-L5, *112,* 115
    level L5-S1, *114,* 118
    level S1-S2, *116,* 118
    level S2-S3, 118
  spinal cord damage, levels L4-S1, 94–95
  tests, level L4, 51, *52, 53*
    level L5, *54, 55,* 57, *59*
    level S1, *58, 59, 60,* 61
    levels S2, S3, S4, 65
    with herniated discs, *68–70*
  inversion, *58*
  plantarflexion, *60*
Forearm, sensation testing, 17, 23
Fractures, cervical spine, 85–88, *85–88*

Gastrocnemius, *60,* 61
  spinal cord lesions, level S1, 95
Gluteal nerve, testing, 61
  at neurologic table levels, 74
Gluteus maximus, *62*
  testing, 61
    in meningomyelocele, *116,* 118, 120–121, *120–121*
Gluteus medius, testing, *57, 59*
  meningomyelocele, level L5-S1, *114*
  and maximus, neurologic levels affecting, table, 74
  spinal cord damage, level L4-S1, 94–95
Grading, of muscle, 2. *See also* Muscle, grading

Hamstrings, neurologic levels affecting, 74
  with meningomyelocele, level L5-S1, *114*
  level S1-S2, 116
  testing, 120, *120*
Hand, motor power, *26,* 27
  with spinal cord lesion, 83
  See also Arm, Fingers
Hangman's fracture, 85, *86*
Heel, muscle testing, 57. *See also,* Foot
Herpes zoster, 71–72
Hip, abduction, *56*
  test, 59
  adductor muscles, neurologic levels affecting, 74
    testing, 49, *50, 51*
  extension, *62*
  flexion, 46–49, *46–49*
    neurologic levels affecting, 74
    with spinal cord damage, levels L1-L5, 94–95
  function, with meningomyelocele, levels L1-L2 and L2-L3, 109
    level L3-L4, *110,* 111
    level L4-L5, *112,* 113
    level L5-S1, *114,* 116–117
    level S1-S2, *116,* 118
    level S2-S3, 118
Hoffmann's sign, 84, *85*
Hydrocephalus, 119
Hydromelia, 119
Hyperextension, neck, 88, *88*
Hyperflexion, neck, 87, *88*
Hyperreflexia, 3
Hyporeflexia, 3

Iliopsoas, function, with meningomyelocele at level L3-L4, 110
  at level L4-L5, *112*
  at level L5-S1, *114*
  at level S1-S2, *116,* 118
  with spinal cord damage, at levels L1-L3, 94
  testing, 46–47, *46–47*
Infrapatellar tendon, reflex, 65
Injuries, spinal, 102, *103,* 104
  spinal cord, 75
Intercostal muscles, testing, 45
Interossei dorsales, 23–25, *24*
  with herniated disc, *32–36*
  in tetraplegia, *78–84*
Interspinous ligament, 101, *101*
Intrinsic muscles, meningomyelocele, *116,* 118

Jefferson fracture, 85, *85*

Knee, extension lag, *48,* 49
 function, with meningomyelocele, 120
   at levels L1-L2, L2-L3, 109
   at level L3-L4, *110,* 111
   at level L4-L5, *112,* 113
   at level L5-S1, *114,* 117
   at level S1-S2, *116,* 118
   at level S2-S3, 118
   with spinal cord damage, at
    levels L4-S1, 94–95
   testing, 47, *48*
    memory aid, *53*
    patellar tendon reflex, 51,
     52, 53

Legs, function, with cord damage,
  levels L1-S1, 94–95
 at neurologic levels L3-S2, 65
 sensation dermatomes, L4 and
  L5, *57,* 59
 and herniated disc, table, 66
 testing scheme, 64–65, *65*
 See also Extremities, lower
Levels, neurologic. *See* Neurologic
  level
Ligamentous complex, posterior,
  101
Ligamentum flavum, 101, *101*
Longitudinal ligament, *30*
 lumbar, *67*
"Low back" pain. *See* Pain
Lumbricals, 21–23, *23*

Median nerve, *14,* 17
 testing, 21–23
Memory aid, C5, biceps reflex, 12
 C6, sensory distribution, *17*
 C8, finger flexors, 23
 L4, patellar tendon reflex, *53, 56*
 L5, toe extensors, *55*
 S1, Achilles tendon reflex, S1, *63*
Meningomyelocele, 107–121
 developmental problems, 118–
  119
 examination of patient, 120
 at level L1-L2, 109
 at level L2-L3, 109
 at level L3-L4, *110, 111,* 111,
  113
 at level L4-L5, *112–113,* 113,
  115–116
 at level L5-S1, *114–115,* 116–
  118
 at level S1-S2 and S2-S3, *117,*
  118
 upper extremity, 119–120
Milestones, of development, 118–
  119
Motion range, chart, *2*

Motor power, evaluation, 1
Motor power tests, with herniated
  discs, *32–36*
 legs, 65
 in meningomyelocele, 108
  in infants, 107
 at neurologic level, C2, with
   spinal cord lesions, *78*
  C3, with spinal cord lesion,
   77–78, *79*
  C4, with spinal cord lesion, 79,
   80
  C5, 7–12, *8*
   with spinal cord lesion, 80,
    81
  C6, 13, *14*
   with spinal cord lesion, 81
  C7, *18*
   with spinal cord lesion, 82
  C8, *22*
   with spinal cord lesion, 83
  T1, 23–25, *24*
   with spinal cord lesion, 83–
    84
  T2 to T12, 45
   with spinal cord lesions, 93
  T12-L3, 47–49, *46–49*
  L1-S1, with spinal cord damage, 94–95
  L3-L4, with meningomyelocele, *110,* 111
  L4, 51, *52*
  L4-L5, with meningomyelocele, *112,* 113, 115
  L5 level, *54,* 57, *57,* 59
  L5-S1, with meningomyelocele, *114,* 116–118
  S1 level, *58*
  S1-S2, with meningomyelocele,
   116, 118
  S2-S3, with meningomyelocele,
   118
  upper extremity, *26,* 27
Motor power. *See also* Muscle
Motorcycles, and nerve root injury,
  42, *43*
Muscles, flaccidity and spasticity,
  97–98
 grading, chart, 2
  cervical, table, 38
  lumbar, table, 66
  thoracic, 100, *100*
 myotomes, 1
 in poliomyelitis, 72–73
 test, extensors of toe, *55*
  of foot, 64
  gastrocnemius-soleus, 61
  gluteus maximus, 61, *62*
  gluteus medius, 59

Muscles, test—(*Continued*)
 of hip adductors, 51
 legs, scheme of, 64
 in meningomyelocele, 120–
  121, *120–121*
 peroneus longus and brevis, *59,*
  61
 sacral sparing, 97, *97*
 wrist extension, *16*
 of trunk and leg, neurologic level
  affecting, 74
Musculocutaneous nerve, *10,* 11,
  17
 testing, 13
 of sensation, 17
Muscle. *See specific muscles. See
  also* Motor power
Myelitis, transverse, 91
Myelogram, of herniated disc, cervical, *37*
 table, 38
 lumbar, *71*
 table, 66
 of meningomyelocele, *108*
Myotome, definition, 1
 electromyogram of, 37

Neck, fractures, 85–88, *85–88*
 spinal cord injuries, 77–92
Nerves, trunk and leg, neurologic
  level affecting, 74
Nerve roots, avulsion of, 42, *43*
 cervical, and herniated disc, 28,
  32–36
  table, 38
 lesions, 5–74
  level C5, 7–12
  C5 to T1, 7–43
  T2 to S4, 45–74
 lumbar, and herniated disc, 66,
  67, *67*
  table, 66
Neurologic level, in meningomyelocele, determination, 107–
  118
 C1-T1, clinical application, 28–
  43
 C2, spinal cord lesion, *78*
 C3, spinal cord lesion, 77–78, *79*
 C4, spinal cord lesion, 78–80, *80*
 C5, herniated disc, *32*
  nerve root testing, 7–12, *8–12*
  spinal cord lesion, 80, *81*
 C6, herniated disc, *33*
  nerve root testing, 13–17, *14*
  spinal cord lesion, 81–82, *82*
 C7, herniated disc, *34*
  nerve root testing, 17–21, *18*
  spinal cord lesion, 82, *83*

Neurologic level—(*Continued*)
  C8, herniated disc, *35*
    nerve root testing, 21–23, *22*
    spinal cord lesion, 83, *84*
    nerve root testing, 23–27, *24*
    spinal cord lesions, 83, *84*
  T1, herniated disc, *36*
  T1-T12, spinal cord lesions, 93
  T1-S2, spinal cord lesions, ambulation, 98
    bladder and bowel control, 98–100
  T2 to T12, testing, 45
  T12-L3, testing, 47–51
  L1-S1, spinal cord damage, 94–95
  L1-S4, related to muscles and nerves, 74
  L1-L2, meningomyelocele, 109
  L2-L3, meningomyelocele, 109
  L3-L4, meningomyelocele, *110–111*, 111, 113
  L3-S1, and poliomyelitis, 73
  L4, disc L3-L4, tests, *68*
    testing, 51–53, 56–57, *52*
  L4-L5, meningomyelocele, *112–113*, 113, 115–116
  L4-S1, clinical application, 68–74
  L4-S1, testing, and back pain, 67
  L5, *54, 55, 56,* 57, 59
    disc L4-L5, tests, *69*
  L5-S1, meningomyelocele, *114–115*, 116–118
  S1, testing, *58,* 61–64
    disc L5-S1, tests, 70
  S1-S2, meningomyelocele, *116–117*, 118
  S2, 3, 4, 64–65
  S2-S3, meningomyelocele, 118
  and spinal cord, 75–121
  upper extremity, 28

Obturator nerve, 49
  neurologic level affecting, 74
Odontoid process, 7
  fracture, 86, *86–87*
Oppenheim's sign, 95, *96*
Osteoarthiritis, cervical spine, table, 38
  tests, 42, *43*
  of uncinate process, 40–42, *41, 43*

P.A.D., palmar interossei, 25
Pain, back, teen-age, 71
  "low back," 67–68
  from herniated disc, 29, 31, *31*
  herpes zoster, 71
  of neck, whiplash, 39–40
  in osteoarthritis, 42–43, *43*
  sensation of, 1–2

Pain—(*Continued*)
  in spondylolysis, 70
Palmar interossei (P.A.D.) testing, 25
Paraplegia, 83–85, 93–96
  ambulation prognostication, 98
  bladder and bowel control, 98–100
Pars interarticularis, *72*
  and spondylolysis, 69
Patellar tendon reflex, *52*
  with herniated lumbar disc, 66, *68–70*
  with herniated thoracic disc, 101
  at L-4 level, 65
  memory aid, *53*
  with meningomyelocele, *111,* 113
  with spinal cord damage, 94–95
Perineum, level affecting, 74
Peroneal nerves, testing, 51, 57, 59, 61
  neurologic levels affecting, 74
Peroneus longus and brevis, *58, 59*
  and herniated discs, 66, *68–70*
  neurologic levels affecting, 65, 74
  testing, 61
Plantar nerves, 74
Poliomyelitis, 72–73
Processes, of vertebra, *40*

Quadriceps, *53*
  with meningomyelocele, L3-L4, *110*
    level L4-L5, *112*
    level L5-S1, *114*
    level S1-S2, *116*
  neurologic levels affecting, 65, 74
  with spinal cord lesions, levels L2-L5, 94–95
  testing, 47–49, *49*
Quadriplegia. *See* Tetraplegia

Radial extensors, 13
Radial nerve, *10, 14, 20,* 21
  testing, 17, *20*
Radiation, of pain. *See* Pain
Rectus abdominus, testing, 45
Rectus femoris, *48*
Reflexes, anal function, 99–100, *100*
  cremasteric, 96, *96*
  with herniated cervical discs, *32–36*
    table, 38
  with herniated lumbar discs, *68–70*
    table, 66
  with herniated thoracic discs, 100–101

Reflexes—(*Continued*)
  with meningomyelocele, levels L1-L2, L2-L3, 109
    level L3-L4, 111, *111,* 113
    level L4-L5, *113,* 116
    level L5-S1, *115,* 118
    level S1-S2, *117,* 118
    level S2-S3, 118
  with spinal cord lesion, level C3, 78, *79*
    level C4, 79–80, *80*
    level C5, 80–81, *81*
    level C6, 82, *82*
    level C7, 82, *83*
    level C8, 83, *84*
    level T1, 84
    levels L1-S1, 94–96, *95–96*
  stretch arc, 2–3
  testing, level C5, biceps tendon, 8, 12, *32*
    level C6, brachioradialis, 13, *14, 16, 33*
    level C7, triceps, *18,* 21, *21,* 34
    level C8, none, *22, 35*
    level T1, none, *24, 36*
    level L4, patellar tendon, 49, 51, *52, 53, 53,* 56
    level L5, none, *54, 59*
    level S1, Achilles tendon, *58,* 61, 63–64, *63*
    levels S2, S3, S4, 64, *64*
  lower extremity, 65
  sacral sparing, 97, *97*
  upper extremity, 27
  in tetraplegia, 84, *78–84*
Respiration, with spinal cord lesions, 78, *78, 79, 79, 80,* 81, 90
Roentgenography, of spine injury, 101, 102, *104*
Roots, of nerves. *See* Nerve root

Sacral sparing, 97–98, *97*
  bladder and bowel control, 99
  in meningomyelocele, 109
Sciatic nerves, 74
Scoliosis, 119
Scotty dog, lumbar spine, *72*
Segments, of spinal cord, 1
Sensation, evaluation methods, 1–2
  with meningomyelocele, level S1-S2, *117,* 118
    levels L1-L2, L2-L3, 109
    level L3-L4, 111, *111*
    level L4-L5, *113,* 115–116
    level L5-S1, *115,* 118
    level S2-S3, 118
  with spinal cord damage, level C5, 80

Sensation, with spinal cord damage
  —(*Continued*)
  level C4, 79, *80*
  level C3, 78
  level T1, 84
  level C8, 83
  level C7, 82
  level C6, 81–82
  levels T1-T12, 93, *94*
  levels L1-S1, 94–95
  in tetraplegia, *78–84*
  testing, arm, 17, 23, 25, 27, *27*
    herniated cervical discs, *32–36,*
      38
    table, 66
  herniated thoracic disc, 100
  legs, scheme of, 64–65
  level C5, axillary nerve, *8,* 12,
    13, 32
  level C6, musculocutaneous
    nerve, *14,* 17, *17, 33*
  level C7, *18,* 21, *34*
  level C8, antebrachial cutane-
    ous nerve, *22,* 23, *35*
  level T1, brachial-cutaneous
    nerve, *24, 25, 36*
  levels T2 to T12, 45, *94*
  levels T12-L3, 49, *50, 51, 51*
  level L4, *52,* 56–57
  level L4-S1, *68–70*
  level L5, *54,* 59
  level S1, *58,* 64
  levels S2, S3, S4, S5, 64
  sacral sparing, 97, *97*
  See also Dermatome
Serratus anterior, testing, 9
Shingles, 71–72
Shock, spinal, 97–98
Shoulder, abduction, 7–9, *8–9*
  spinal cord damage, level C5, 80
  level C6, 81
Sitting, development, 118
Skin, dermatomes, 1
Soleus, *60, 61*
  spinal cord lesions, level S1,
    95
Spasticity, of muscles, 97–98
Spinal cord, bifid, 119
  lesions, 75–121
    cervical, 77–92
      level C2, *78*
      level C3, 77–78, *79*
      level C4, 79–80, *80*
      level C5, 80–81, *81*
      level C-6, 81–82, *82*
      level C7, 82–83, *83*
      level C8, 83, *84*
    clinical application, 96–101
    complete or incomplete, 96–
      97, 99–100

Spinal cord, lesions—(*Continued*)
  lumbar, level L1, L2, L3, 94
    level L4, 94–95
    level L5, S1, 95
  thoracic, level T1, 83–84
    levels T1–T12, 93–105
  protection following, 101–102,
    104–105
  in poliomyelitis, 72, *73*
  segments of, 1
Spinal shock, 97–98
  after trauma, 77
Spine, cervical, articulation, *29*
  fractures, 85–88, *85–88*
  sprain, 39–40
  tests for osteoarthritis, 42, *43*
  fusion, 102
  injury, compression, 104, 105
    flexion, 102, *103,* 104
    flexion-rotation, 102, *103,* 104,
      105
    hyperextension, 104, 105
  stability after injury, 101–105
    criteria for, cervical section,
      102
    thoracolumbar and lumbar
      sections, 105
  thoracic and lumbar, *99*
Spinothalamic tracts, 1–2, *2*
Spinous process, of vertebra, *40*
Spondylolysis, 68–71, *72*
Spondylolysthesis, 68–71
Sprain, cervical neck, 39–40
Stability of spine, 101–105
Standing, development, 118–119
Stretch reflex. *See* Reflex, stretch
Suprascapular nerve, 8–9, *8*
Supraspinous ligament, 101, *101*
Supraspinatus, testing, 9
Syringomyelia, 120

Temperature, sensation of, 1–2
Test, Valsalva, cervical discs, 39
  distraction, of osteoarthritis, 42,
    43
  See also Muscle testing, Sensory
    testing, Reflex testing
Testing, in meningomyelocele, 120–
  121, *120–121*
Tetraplegia, 77–92
  level C2, *78*
  level C3, *79*
Tibial nerves, levels affecting, 74
Tibialis anterior, testing, 51, *52, 53,*
  65
  for herniated discs, *68–70*
  table, 66
  with meningomyelocele, level L4-
    L5, *112,* 115
  level L5-S1, *114*

Tibialis anterior—(*Continued*)
  with spinal cord lesions, levels,
    L4-L5, 94–95
  and posterior, 74
Toes, clawed, 64
  extensors, memory aid, *55*
    at neurologic levels, 65
    testing, 57, 59
  intrinsic muscles, 74
  with spinal cord damage, 95
  tests of, *55*
Touch, sensation of, 2
Transverse foramen, 7
Transverse process, cervical spine, 7
Triceps, tendon reflex, *18,* 21, *21,*
  27
  herniated disc, *32–36*
  spinal cord damage, 82
  in tetraplegia, *78–84*
  testing, 17–*18*
Trunk, nerve root lesions, 45–74
Tuberculosis, cervical spine, 91
Tumors, cervical spine, 91

Ulnar extensors, 13
Ulnar nerve, *14,* 17, 20
  testing, 21–25, *24*
Uncinate process, and herniated
    discs, table, 38
  and osteoarthritis, *40,* 40–42

Valsalva test, 39
Vastus lateralis, 48
Vastus medialis, *48–49*
Vertebrae, cervical, 28
  anatomy of, *40*
  fracture, 85–88, *85–88*
  facet joint dislocation, 88–90,
    88–90
  lumbar, *67–70, 72*
  slippage of, 68–69
  thoracic and lumbar, *99*
  See also Spine

Walking, development, 119
Wheelchair, spinal cord lesions, 80,
  81, 82, 84, 90
  See also Ambulation
Whiplash injury, 39–40, *39*
Wink, anal, reflex. *See* Anal reflex
Wrist, extension, test, C6, *14*
  extensors, testing, 13–17, *14–16*
    herniated disc, *32–36*
    spinal cord damage, 81
    and flexors, in tetraplegia, *78–*
      84
  flexion test, *18,* 20
  flexors, 17–21, *19, 20*
    with herniated disc, *32–36*
    with spinal cord damage, 82